NURSES ON THE MOVE

A VOLUME IN THE SERIES

The Culture and Politics of Health Care Work
EDITED BY SUZANNE GORDON AND SIOBAN NELSON

Code Green: Money-Driven Hospitals and the Dismantling of Nursing
Dana Weinberg

Nobody's Home: Candid Reflections of a Nursing Home Aide
Thomas Edward Gass

Nursing against the Odds: How Health Care Cost Cutting, Media Stereotypes, and Medical Hubris Undermine Nurses and Patient Care
Suzanne Gordon

NURSES ON THE MOVE

Migration and the Global Health Care Economy

Mireille Kingma

ILR Press
AN IMPRINT OF
CORNELL UNIVERSITY PRESS
ITHACA AND LONDON

First published 2006 by Cornell University Press
First printing, Cornell Paperbacks, 2006

Printed in the United States of America

Library of Congress Cataloging-in-Publication Data

Kingma, Mireille.
  Nurses on the move : migration and the global health care economy / Mireille Kingma.
    p. cm. — (The culture and politics of health care work)
Includes bibliographical references and index.
  ISBN-13: 978-0-8014-4305-3 (cloth : alk. paper)
  ISBN-10: 0-8014-4305-9 (cloth : alk. paper)
  ISBN-13: 978-0-8014-7259-6 (pbk. : alk. paper)
  ISBN-10: 0-8014-7259-8 (pbk. : alk. paper)
  1. Nurses, Foreign. 2. Nurses—Supply and demand.
I. Title. II. Series.
  [DNLM: 1. Transcultural Nursing. 2. Foreign Professional Personnel. 3. Nursing—manpower.
4. Career Mobility.
WY 107 K54n 2006]
  RT89.3.K56 2006
  331.12′91362173—dc22   2005018420

Cornell University Press strives to use environmentally responsible suppliers and materials to the fullest extent possible in the publishing of its books. Such materials include vegetable-based, low-VOC inks and acid-free papers that are recycled, totally chlorine-free, or partly composed of nonwood fibers. For further information, visit our website at www.cornellpress.cornell.edu.

Cloth printing   10 9 8 7 6 5 4 3 2 1
Paperback printing   10 9 8 7 6 5 4 3 2 1

To Mom—for her courage and passionate interest in the world around her,

To Stuart—for his love, companionship, and unfailing support,

To Alexandre, Hope, and Brooke—for the joy they bring.

Contents

Acknowledgments

The time and expertise of many people go into making a book. The subject of nurse migration touches a wide range of disciplines, industries, and organizations as well as people. I have been very fortunate, benefiting from the gracious sharing of data, personal experiences, and professional analysis by friends and colleagues as well as by new acquaintances willing to be interviewed. To all of them I cannot sufficiently express my gratitude for their generous and valuable contributions.

Organizations that have provided a wealth of information and technical support include the World Health Organization, the International Labour Organization, the International Organization for Migration, the World Trade Organization, the Commonwealth Secretariat, and, of course, the International Council of Nurses. Special thanks go to Judith Oulton, Christine Hancock, Jean-Guy Carrier, Peggy Vidot, Barbara Stilwell, Danielle Grondin, Christiane Wiskow, and Piyasiri Wickramasekara. Appreciation also needs to be expressed to Tim Martineau (Liverpool School of Tropical Medicine) for the kind sharing of knowledge and documentation.

National organizations such as the Royal College of Nursing (UK), the Swedish Association of Health Professionals, the Korean Nurses Association, the Democratic Nursing Organization of South Africa, the Panama Nurses Association, the Samoa Nurses Association, the Mauritius Nursing Association, the American Nurses Association, the Canadian Nurses Association, UNISON, the Royal College of Nursing (Australia), and the Philippine Nurses Association (including the PNA of America) have been particularly helpful in connecting me with nurses who have experienced the advantages and disadvantages of migration. I am grateful to Lolita Compas and Judy Sheridan-Gonzalez of the New York State Nurses Association for facilitating access to migrant staff nurses and providing the perspective of a professional nurses' union in the United States. Ellen Sanders and Barbara Nichols from the Commission on Graduates of Foreign Nursing Schools, Joe Nichols from the Nursing and Midwifery Council, and Paul de Raeve from the Standing Committee of Nurses in the European Union have been particularly helpful in clarifying the professional credentialing of foreign-educated nurses in the United States, the United Kingdom, and the European Union—their contributions are greatly appreciated.

This book would have remained faceless without the personal stories of the many nurses I interviewed. Their life experiences provide depth and voice to this discussion of nurse migration. While many remain anonymous in this book, I remember each one and admire their courage and determination to seek a better life for themselves and their families.

I thank Cornell University Press, especially Fran Benson, editorial director, and Suzanne Gordon and Sioban Nelson, series coeditors, for the trust and support they gave throughout the development of this book. It has been an incredible adventure and learning experience. Suzanne Gordon's excellent communication and mentoring skills have greatly contributed to the final product. Her enthusiasm and thought-provoking questions created a positive environment where work became fun and progress was inevitable. I have come to admire John LeRoy's skill with words. His copy editor's magic transformed a manuscript into a book. Thanks also go to Kay Banning for her excellent work in creating a comprehensive and user-friendly index.

Last but not least, I would like to thank you, the reader, for your interest in exploring the many obscure as well as obvious facets of nurse migration—a significant social phenomenon that provides insight on the increasing mobility of professional workers and has a major impact on the global health care economy.

Introduction

I have always been a migrant. Soon after I was born in my grandparents' home in the French-speaking part of Switzerland, my mother took me to German-speaking Zurich where she and my father had recently settled. At a very young age, I was already an internal or intranational migrant, embarking on my first cultural and linguistic adventure. When I turned four, my father became an international economic migrant, and I found myself sailing across the Atlantic with my parents and brother to the United States. There, equipped with a green card and the status of alien, or permanent resident, I spent the better part of eighteen years in New York City. Educated in the United States, but with deep roots in my homeland, I traveled back to Europe for my first work experiences as a professional nurse. I worked in Switzerland, then moved for several years to the United Kingdom, and from there went on to Spain. After I married and had a child, I returned to Switzerland, certain that my traveling days were over. Little did I know that they had only just begun.

In 1984 I joined the staff of the International Council of Nurses (ICN), an international federation of national nurses' associations from 126 countries. Over the years I have exchanged ideas, trained, and been trained in more than sixty countries; I have flown around the world numerous times and have been enriched by the exposure to different perspectives, cultures, societies, and health systems. I have had the privilege of working with nurses from all over the world—some of them nationals, some of them migrants. Many of these nurses have shared their life experiences with me and confided their hopes as well as their fears, both professional and personal. Their stories have touched me and strengthened my commitment as an advocate for social justice.

Within the ICN secretariat, I carry major responsibility for one of the organization's three main activity areas—the Socio-Economic Welfare Program, which focuses on the pay, working conditions, and work environment of nurses. International trade in services, occupational health and safety, and human resources management are central to my work. Naturally, nurse migration has become an important element of my portfolio. This has led to close contact and cooperation with colleagues in other international organizations, such as the World Health Organization, the International Labour Organization, the World Trade Organization, and the International Organization for Migration. In the light of today's massive and global nurse migration, it is not surprising that nurses and nursing are at center stage of international debate and discussion.

The implications of migration can be deeply personal and complex. Indeed it is becoming an intimate fact of life for millions of patients and caregivers all across the globe. No country today is untouched by nurse migration. A staggering number of nurses worldwide—the vast majority of them women—are searching for better pay and working conditions, career mobility, professional development, a better life, personal safety, or sometimes just novelty and adventure. They form an important tributary feeding the vast sea of 192 million migrants covering the world today.

The results of this migration can be witnessed in major city hospitals in London, New York, Sydney, or Geneva as well as in Johannesburg, Dakar, Bangkok, or Santiago. The patients come from every possible race, religion, and ethnic background, and the people who take care of them represent an ever-greater kaleidoscope of nationalities—Finnish nurses are treating West Indians in London, South African nurses staff hospitals in Saudi Arabia, a Filipino nurse works in a rural Icelandic hospital. In Switzerland the nurses' French may be tinged with the charm of a Québecois accent, whereas in Melbourne their English may be peppered with New Zealand intonations and slang.

While nursing has been advertised as a "portable profession" and nurses have always moved from town to town, city to city, and country to country, never has nurse migration been the mass phenomenon we see today. Foreign-educated health professionals represent more than a quarter of the medical and nursing workforces of Australia, Canada, the United Kingdom, and the United States.[1] In the Philippines, an average of 2,600 people leave daily for overseas work, and one estimate puts the total number of Philippine-exported nurses at 250,000.[2] In 2001 more Zimbabwean nurses were registered in the United Kingdom than were trained in Zimbabwe that year.[3] In Switzerland 30 percent of employed registered nurses are foreign educated, and in one university hospital 70 percent of new recruits are from abroad.[4] In 2002 the number of foreign-educated nurse entrants to the UK

Nursing and Midwifery Council Register exceeded the number of newly qualified nurses educated in the United Kingdom.[5] Similarly, two-thirds of the new entrants to the Irish nursing register were from other European Union (EU) and international sources, for example, the United Kingdom, Philippines, Australia, South Africa, and India.[6] In parts of the United States and the United Kingdom, it is not unusual to find that internationally recruited nurses make up 60–70 percent of the total number of employed nurses in a given health facility.

Nurse migration is now a widely publicized and major issue, with profound ethical, social, economic, and, of course, health implications. It is considered by many to be the solution of choice to a critical shortage of nurses, whose magnitude threatens health systems around the world.

Patients expect that nurses will be there to respond to their needs, protect them from risk, and help them recover. But there are just not enough nurses available to do the job. A survey conducted by the American Hospital Association found that among the 1,501 responding hospitals, 62 percent of them (75 percent of urban hospitals and 91 percent of all hospitals with over three hundred beds) reported being at or over operating capacity. One-third of all hospitals had experienced "emergency department diversion," that is, refused admission to patients arriving by ambulance. The most common reason was lack of staffed critical care beds; at least 20 percent of the time these hospitals experienced registered nurse vacancy rates of 16 percent.[7] Similarly, in Western Australia "patients were left in emergency department corridors for up to two days before being admitted and there had been at least six cases during the month when all three teaching hospitals had asked to go on ambulance diversion at the same time."[8] The chief medical officer identified the chronic shortage of nurses as the cause of the chaos and inability to provide care.

The way many health services today deal with the nursing shortage breeds international recruitment and migration, which in turn may exacerbate shortages in the countries of origin. Instead of developing a strategic plan to retain their nurses by paying them more and giving them adequate working conditions and authority within their institutions, hospitals and health care systems play a numbers game with the expanding international labor market—a strange version of musical chairs where there are always more empty seats than players. Indeed, the mad scramble for nurses dramatically globalizes the health-sector labor market and encourages international recruitment as a solution to domestic or institutional problems. At the same time, nurses may find that the only way they can advance professionally or solve their workplace, security, and personal problems is by emigrating.

What was recently labeled as a short-term solution to the nursing short-age is now widely recognized as a permanent dimension of human resources management to ensure safe staffing. Today, mass recruitment campaigns have greatly enhanced the opportunities and incentives for nurses to migrate. In addition, recent legislation, trade agreements, and economic policies have facilitated nurse migration. The heightened competition for available nurs-ing human resources, both within and among countries, is generating un-regulated international recruitment practices on a scale without precedent.

Because nurse migration now exists at such a massive pitch, creating equally significant losses and gains, it is imperative to document the social and economic framework and impact of international recruitment, the cur-rent employment practices, and the daily realities of migrant nurses. Clearly, this task is long overdue. To reach an understanding of these complex phe-nomena requires both a study of current health care planning and an in-depth look at the promises and challenges of globalization. Nurses are largely female, and my research confirms a widely acknowledged trend— the feminization of migration patterns. My use of the pronoun *she* to refer to nurses reflects the predominance of women in the profession globally and facilitates the expression of ideas, but used generically it denotes male nurses as well.

This book attempts to present the nature of nurse migration using con-crete examples taken from a wide range of countries offering typical and noteworthy atypical characteristics. Not all countries appear in the book, but readers everywhere should be able to relate to the examples provided. While different categories of nursing personnel exist, the focus will be on the pro-fessional or registered nurse.

Nurse migration illuminates how the rapid changes associated with glob-alization not only offer welcome signs of progress but give rise to dilemmas that can undermine health care. While some advocates of globalization promise that mass migration will lead to economic progress, others worry that these changes threaten a sustainable development of health care systems.

Nurse migration is a multifaceted and intricate social phenomenon. It represents part of the solution for some countries, health systems, or indi-viduals, part of the problem for others. Determining whether nurse migra-tion is more promise than problem is particularly important, not least because the impact of the globalization of the nursing workforce falls largely on the ill and vulnerable human beings whom nurses serve.

This book explores the questions and challenges generated by interna-tional nurse mobility. Chapter 1 looks at the numbers—the statistics that re-veal the extent of nurse migration today. It presents a taxonomy that helps us understand the different categories of nurse migrants and why they migrate. Given the same situation, why does one nurse decide to stay and another to leave? Do we have the tools to predict the size and direction of migration flows? In this chapter, I introduce two main concepts that make massive nurse migration possible: *push* and *pull* factors. These are the conditions and environments that drive nurses out of their home countries and the factors that draw them toward another. I also discuss why the global nursing shortage exists. What factors are at work in the industrialized and developing countries? When did this acute shortage generate the aggressive international recruitment campaigns seen today?

The awesome numbers of nurses needed around the globe tend to make us forget that we are dealing with individuals with their own knowledge and sets of skills, attitudes, and motivations. In fact, many discussions and policies regulating the international mobility of workers—for example, the General Agreement on Trade in Services (GATS)—seem to dehumanize the very human beings that make up the migrant stream. In bureaucratese, migrants are no longer people, workers, or human resources but are referred to as "natural persons" (as distinct from "juridical persons," i.e., enterprises and other legal entities). One has to wonder if this is an attempt to dehumanize people or, the reverse, to humanize commercial entities?

Chapter 2 goes beyond the statistics so that we can understand why nurses leave their countries and what they find when they reach their destination. Here I further explore a fundamental question of this book: Is migration a matter of choice or is it imposed on nurses as an obligation or constraint? For many nurses, migration may seem to be a matter of free will. Yet, when we delve deeply, we see that social and economic conditions in their homelands may practically oblige them to abandon their homes and families to find employment abroad. Moreover, nurse migrants, their families, and their communities may pay a high social cost for this "choice." What does it mean to a society, a community, a family, when, as in the Philippines, 250,000 nurses leave their country—and for most of them this means leaving their parents, their siblings, their husbands, their children—to work abroad? What happens to these children, the future generation? And finally, what welcome is reserved for migrant nurses? After they have been aggressively recruited, what will be the quality of their new social environment and work life? And how will their managers and colleagues treat them?

Large-scale nurse recruitment has another important dimension. It offers endless opportunities for business ventures. Chapter 3 considers the huge opportunity for profit and gain that nurse migration brings to a variety of entrepreneurs. Concern for profit and economic survival also informs the new entrepreneurialism of academic institutions, licensing bodies, and governments. Today, small and big businesses alike are interested in the potential of nurse migration. The health care sector is among the most rapidly growing sectors in the world economy. In the Organisation for Economic Cooperation and Development countries alone it generates approximately $3 trillion per year, incentive enough to attract quite a number of entrepreneurs.[9] These include not only conventional businesses like recruitment agencies and travel agents but also some less likely ones such as schools of nursing, nursing organizations and publishers, and even banks and telephone companies.

No discussion of the economics of nurse migration can exclude a look at its impact on countries from which nurses migrate. Migrant workers send money home to their families. Remittances sent through formal banks, post offices, or financial institutions total an estimated 75–200 billion dollars per year. In some countries, this represents a substantial percentage of their gross domestic product: for example, 4.5 percent in Benin, 5.8 percent in Burkina Faso, 16.2 percent in Nicaragua, and 26.5 percent in Lesotho. If savings sent to families informally is included, the total sum doubles or in some cases triples. Remittances are substantially higher than the total funds made available by overseas development agencies. In Africa, with the exception of Nigeria and Cameroon, remittances account for considerably more than foreign direct investment and are thus an essential contribution to the national economy. They constitute a key source of global finance and must be included in the migration debate.

The scope of the for-profit economic activity and the potential for exploitation of nurse migrants has created great concern and activity in the trade unions and professional organizations representing nurses. Can existing institutions guarantee migrants an environment free from abuse and discrimination?

To deal with nurse migration, countries and governmental bodies have set up regional, national, and international commissions, proposed or implemented regulations, issued ethical statements, and even tried to enact bans limiting migration. When we examine the national and international responses to nurse migration closely, we discover many double standards and vested interests involved in policy decisions and declarations issued by policy makers, politicians, health system administrators, and organizations. Chapter 4 explores the many ironies and contradictions in the discussions, debates, and attempts to develop policies around nurse migration. For example, although Nelson Mandela specifically requested the United Kingdom in 1999 to stop recruiting nurses from South Africa, his country was then employing physicians from neighboring countries. Notably, 78 percent of the rural physicians in South Africa were not nationals at the time.

Various attempts have been made to provide guidelines that dissuade (not outlaw) abusive recruitment practices targeting developing countries faced with critical nursing shortages. When examining this issue, again questions abound. How can migration be controlled or managed without infringing upon individuals' freedom of movement and exposing the recruitment process to even greater corruption and double standards? How can we maintain the delicate balance between the human and labor rights of the individual and a collective concern for the health of a nation's population? Who is negotiating the framework for the global movement of nurses? The term *negotiation* immediately implies a set of stakeholders or concerned parties. What are the vested interests behind nurse migration? Where is the financial and social gain?

The morass of policy proposals and position statements seems to pale in complexity when one considers the intricate and often convoluted web of legislation, trade agreements, and economic policies that are negotiated on an international level to support international nurse mobility. In chapter 5 we will look at the baffling array of global rules and regulations upon which migration depends. In this chapter as in others, questions of professional regulation resurface—definitions of just who is a nurse, what education is required, and how qualifications are verified. What are the labor, immigration, and licensing terms of reference that govern nurse migration?

A final set of questions emerges in relation to nurse migration. These are embedded in the brain-drain/brain-gain debates that are ever present when shortages and migration are linked, inevitably leading to heated and defensive discussion. Is the migration solution to shortages efficient, or are we wasting precious resources? What mechanisms are in place to protect the vulnerable from exploitation and abuse? Where are the pros and cons of migration, and what consequences ensue when the pros gain the advantage?

Increasingly, migration is seen as a means for development and a better distribution of global wealth. Migration may, however, be a path to economic advancement mainly in mid- and high-income countries where individuals have better access to education, training, communication services, and transport. Nurse mobility could potentially improve *or* reduce access to quality health services. While some developing countries are hemorrhaging from nurse migration, others are benefiting from exchange programs, and still others find migration a solution to high unemployment levels. Nurse migration is a mirror reflecting the positive and the negative—it expresses what exists behind the numbers. For the individual nurse, migration may be either a chance for a better life or a sentence to a nightmarish existence. For an ailing health care sector, nurse migrants can be the rescue or condemn it to failure.

Brain drain, brain gain, and what has been called "brain circulation" are all possible scenarios that result from nurse migration. It is, however, imperative to understand that a growing reliance of major health systems in industrialized countries on nurses recruited from abroad threatens the sustainability of services at the cutting edge of science and referral sites for the rest of the world. International recruitment is costly and grossly unreliable. At any moment, recruited nurses can return to their homeland or migrate to another country if better conditions are offered. The source of recruited nurses in a given country may dry up and no other pool of nurses found to take its place. The international labor market evolves, responding to world events and fluctuating socioeconomic factors. Continuity of care, a needed dimension of health services to the population, is put at risk when a critical mass of personnel is undergoing constant turnover.

In the conclusion of this book, I look at some of the assumptions that create the conditions that fuel nurse migration—the idea, for example, that a nurse is a nurse is a nurse. I suggest critical areas for further research and present strategies that enhance the positive and reduce the negative effects of international nurse migration.

The available statistics clearly indicate that a dangerous nursing shortage will continue for at least another ten to twenty years. While administrators may consider international migration to be a way to assure safe staffing, I will argue that it is in fact a symptom of the larger systemic problems that make nurses leave their jobs and the countries in which they work. Is migration really the root of the problem? Shouldn't we be addressing the need to migrate, which is systematically being obscured by diversionary slogans and extreme posturing? Although some nurses migrate only to seek adventure, too many, as we will see, do so because they cannot find a safe haven or decent working conditions anywhere in their country of origin. Migration may indeed be a free choice on their part, but it is a choice that many make because of the constraints in the workplace or the broader society. Since nurse migration will be with us for a long time to come, it is critical to learn as much as possible about its driving forces, participants, stakeholders, and impact.

1. Welcome to Globalization

"I feel safe. I am happy here and can now plan my life."

Fatima Ansari*, the nurse I am talking to in Stockholm, is a trim, well-dressed woman in her mid-thirties with dark eyes that communicate calm and strength. She was born in the Middle East, member of an ethnic community representing only 7 percent of the national population. Life was difficult but she grew up in a happy home, sheltered by her immediate and extended family. Ansari dreamed of being a nurse, but making the wish a reality was a continuing challenge. Women were expected to marry young, care for their husbands, and immediately build families. In spite of the powerful social pressures, Ansari persevered and with the support of her parents finished nursing school. What a momentous occasion, the day she received her diploma! It came with the promise of a wonderful future.

In her first job Ansari faced what would become an insurmountable obstacle. The fact that she belonged to an ethnic minority made her the butt of intolerable discrimination. In the eleven years Ansari worked as a nurse in her home country, she was never given a permanent position and was daily victimized by the harmful and unfair practices of her colleagues and employers. Eager to pursue her nursing education, she made countless unsuccessful attempts to enroll in continuing education courses and advanced university programs. Despite her qualifications and willingness to learn, she was consistently refused admittance. Earning very little money and only offered sporadic temporary work contracts, she often had to work more than one job to make ends meet. Despite all her efforts, a permanent position, professional fulfillment, and career advancement became an illusion. Every day she felt more insecure and unsafe. Unable to plan her life, she was at the

---

* An asterisk following a name indicates a pseudonym.

mercy of her employers and bullied by her colleagues. As she grew older and remained single, her career ambitions isolated her more every day.

Ansari knew that in her country there was a serious nursing shortage. Seeing the desperate need for nurses made her job insecurities and poor working conditions that much more stressful and difficult to bear. Given no hope of a better future in her home country, Ansari finally decided to join her sister and brother in Sweden. "Moving to Sweden has been a positive experience, and I have been treated well—better than in my home country," she insists. "The decision to move was mine and I would do it again."

Vicki Bigambo* also faced serious professional and personal problems in her home country of Tanzania. A recruitment agency convinced her that she would find a better life if she went to Glasgow to work for a private nursing home. Upon arrival she found quite the opposite. The recruiter had led her to believe that the home was in the heart of the city. In fact, it was located a hundred miles out of town. Bigambo had been promised a salary of £16,000 per year and told that her travel costs would be covered. She was, however, never reimbursed for her travel expenses of over £1,000.

As to the salary, once in Scotland, agency representatives informed her that if she wanted to stay, she would have to sign a new contract for £11,000 per year, even though she was fully responsible for the one-hundred-bed home and was entitled to a much higher salary. Bigambo was asked to give up her passport and warned that if she spoke to anyone about her situation she would be deported.[1]

International Migration

Fatima Ansari and Vicki Bigambo are part of the growing tide of international migrant workers whose rising numbers are one of the most reliable indicators of the rapid rate of globalization. Every country today is affected by international migration, whether as a country of origin, destination, transit, or all three.

Since 1970, the number of international migrants has more than doubled. The increase has kept pace with that of the world's population (from three to six billion people over approximately the same period). The average global annual flow of both temporary and permanent migration has continued to increase over the past decade. According to the International Organization for Migration (IOM), if all international migrants lived in the same place they would constitute the world's fifth-biggest country. In 2004 as many as 192 million people—the equivalent of the entire population of Brazil or Indonesia—moved around the globe. Of the 9 billion people that are predicted to inhabit the world in 2050, there will be some 230 million migrants.[2]

Today, at the start of the twenty-first century, one out of every thirty-five persons worldwide is an international migrant. Some 48 percent of these migrants are women, an indication of the rising feminization of migration patterns. Women migrants are becoming agents of economic change for many countries as they enter the international labor market.[3]

A common assumption is that women and men moving from developing to more industrialized countries largely drive international migration. In fact, 60 percent of migrants were absorbed by the Western industrialized nations in 2000. One out of every ten persons in industrialized countries is an international migrant. Indeed, the very nature of national populations is changing as a result of global mobility.

Most of the people who move across the globe are motivated by professional or occupational concerns or are family members accompanying the migrant worker. The International Labour Organization (ILO) tells us there are an estimated eighty-one million international migrant workers in the world. If one focuses only on highly skilled migration, the United States, Japan, and Canada have recently had the largest annual inflows, totaling 585,200 persons. Yet in the same time period, another 80,800 professional workers moved to the United Kingdom, Australia, and Germany.[4] It is difficult to imagine a population the size of Boston arriving in Canada or Japan every single year.

Migration is often believed to be a phenomenon bred by extreme poverty or political chaos. Yet the migration of highly skilled workers represents an increasingly large component of total migration. It is estimated that 1.5 million professionals from developing countries work in industrialized countries.[5] Physicians and nurses are part of this professional migration stream.

International nurse migration is not a new phenomenon. In the 1960s and 1970s it was not unusual for new graduates from Australia and New Zealand to travel through North America and Europe for a year's working holiday. In 1970 more Filipino nurses were registered in the United States and Canada than in the Philippines.[6] Today, however, the flow of nurse migration is changing dramatically because a wider range of supplier countries is satisfying the growing labor needs of industrialized countries. For example, the number of countries sending international nurse recruits to the United Kingdom has increased from seventy-one in 1990 to ninety-five in 2001.[7]

Although the focus of this book is global nurse migration, it is important to understand that the migrant stream, like a river flowing into a vast sea, is fed by tributaries. The first step on the international migration journey is often intranational migration. Nurses may move from rural to urban areas or from the public to the private sector within a country. They may move from the health *care* sector to the wider health industry, for example, from a hospital to a pharmaceutical company. Or they may quit the health system and take up employment in areas such as clothing retail. Stretching the definition of migration, nurses may also migrate right out of the labor market, when they take a career break or early retirement.

Internal migrants may represent a significant pool of nurses. It is often argued that the exodus of nurses from the public to the private health sector harms those patients who depend on public services, which are usually cheaper or free. In spite of its importance, internal nurse migration tends to elude currently available statistics. When it comes to public-sector health workforce data, the statistics are often unavailable, patchy, no longer current, or even contradictory.[8] It is even harder to determine the number of nurses working in the private sector. Although the distinction between internal and international migration is important if universal health care coverage of the population is to be planned and achieved, there are no reliable monitoring systems in place to compare the loss of nurses from the public health service through internal as opposed to international migration.

Available documents and anecdotal reports clearly indicate that when nurses run out of intranational options, they opt for global mobility. The mass migration that is happening today is not only greater in magnitude than past migrant patterns, it is also different in its direction and location. Traditionally, international nurse migration tended to be a North–North phenomenon. For example, Irish nurses went to the United Kingdom or Canadian nurses sought higher pay in the United States. South–South migration is, however, also a common phenomenon and highlights regional recruitment patterns with, for example, nurses from Fiji working in Palau, South African nurses working in the Seychelles, and Cuban nurses recruited to Nicaragua. While much of the international flow of nurses is from one industrialized country to another, and a substantial share is relatively short term, it is the recent and rapid growth in international recruitment from developing countries that has gained most media and policy attention.

There has been a major focus on South–North migration as more Ghanaian nurses move to the United Kingdom, Vietnamese nurses work in France, and Indian and Chinese nurses are recruited to Ireland. In 2000 over five hundred nurses left Ghana for employment in the industrialized countries. That number was more than twice the number of new graduates from nursing programs in the country that year.[9] In Malawi, between 1999 and 2001 over 60 percent of the entire staff of registered nurses in a single tertiary hospital (114 nurses) left for employment in other countries.[10] In Jamaica 95 percent of the training output of nurses between 1978 and 1985 was lost to international migration, most of which involved employment in industrialized countries.[11]

Some nurses take an indirect route to their final destination, using stops along the way to build up their skills and credentials. For example, a nurse may move from Ghana to the United Kingdom, then head to Canada only to leave one or two years later for what is often the ultimate destination, the United States. Or her route may be even more circuitous, starting in India with stops in Saudi Arabia, the United Kingdom, and then North America. Forty percent of the Filipino nurses working in the United Kingdom have previously worked in Southeast Asia and the Middle East.[12] This duplicates the "carousel" movement of physicians that is already widely acknowledged.[13]

Most countries do not collect data on who migrates, the migrants' motives, or the length of stay abroad.[14] But from interviews and discussions with nurses, it is clear that not all nurses aim for what has been considered to be the carousel's golden ring, work in a highly industrialized country like the United States. Some nurses want to enter industrialized countries so that they can gain education and experience in a particular nursing specialty like oncology or critical care. Once they have enhanced their skills and broadened their knowledge, many of these nurses return to the developing world, either their country of origin or another, to serve populations in desperate need.

Motivations for Migration

To understand the scope and complexity of nurse migration, it is important to know not only where nurses move but why they move. Although migration theory has been evolving for many decades, determining why nurses migrate is a complex matter, and no one theory has yet captured all the forces that influence an individual's decision to move.

Traditionally, migration was thought to occur when "the present value of wages in the destination country exceeded the present value of wages in the source country by more than the direct costs of migration and the preference for remaining at home."[15] In other words, when the perceived cost of moving is less than the perceived cost of staying, migration will take place. This economic theory does not, however, explain why migration occurs even in the absence of wage incentives. The salary scales of US staff nurses tend to be the highest in the world. But many of these nurses are also on the move, both within and out of the United States. Traditional economic theory does not help us understand why relatively highly paid nurses are found working in other countries for less pay. It is obvious that other factors are at play.

According to Dr. Marko Vujicic, a World Bank health economist, salaries are a key factor influencing the supply of migrants, although not the only factor. Even when the earnings are adjusted for purchasing power, the nurse wage in Australia and Canada is about twenty-five times the nurse wage in Zambia, fourteen times the nurse wage in Ghana, and about twice the nurse wage in South Africa. If wages were the decisive factor, it would be logical that more Ghanaian nurses than South African nurses would migrate to an industrialized country because the rewards would be that much greater. In reality, the proportion of health workers who intend to emigrate from South Africa is approximately equal to that in Ghana, suggesting once again that other factors beyond pay influence workers' decisions.[16]

Migration experts increasingly recognize the strong influence of diasporas, currently referred to as transnational communities. As well as other factors like political forces, poverty, and the age of the migrant, past colonial and cultural ties and an existing émigré population in the destination country will play a significant role in the decision to migrate. The migrant's desire to reunite with family and the indirect social costs of migration are weighed against each other. When asked why they migrated, many nurses speak about the encouragement received from relatives or friends already living and working in the destination country. This connection not only stimulated or reinforced their desire to migrate but facilitated access to information, work permits, and employment.

In fact, successful past emigration tends to encourage more future emigration. The more people who have migrated from the source country to the destination country, the greater will be the quantity of information sent back. As a result, there tends to be an increase in this flow of migrants. Such migration, sometimes referred to as "chain migration," often makes the social transition easier for the migrant.[17] Networks of the diaspora also provide financial support for travel. If the nurse is asked to go through a training period to upgrade her skills, for which she may receive little or no wages, the support of friends or relatives will be critical. Such assistance is frequently offered as repayment for what they received as new migrants. If family members are part of the diaspora, this financial and social support may represent their active participation in a family decision or investment.[18]

Despite the obvious wage differentials between high- and low-income countries, it is interesting that few nurses tend to migrate from the very poor countries.[19] When their circumstances are too dire, the constraints they face seem insurmountable. They cannot get credit to finance their move, and they have poor access to information about employment opportunities abroad.

This situation may, however, be changing as aggressive recruitment agencies spread their nets further to find new source countries and offer more comprehensive recruitment packages covering expenses for accreditation, travel, and accommodation.

With so many millions of nurses on the move, it would be impossible to present a complete taxonomy of their goals and motivations. But certain categories do emerge, although any given migrant may fall within more than one category or change from one to another.

Let us start with permanent migration. Since one of the most important motivations is financial, the *economic migrant* is perhaps the largest category of international nurse migrant. The economic migrant is attracted by a better standard of living or by the possibility that she can provide additional income for family members who remain behind in the source country. Sometimes this latter motivation is so important that nurses actually accept a lower standard of living in the destination country in order to send a greater percentage of their income back to the family. In countries, like India, where more than 50 percent of the nurses are unemployed, finding employment in a foreign country may be the only way to earn a living wage and meet the financial needs of the family.

The *quality-of-life migrant* is more interested in questions of safety and well-being. They may be distinguished from economic migrants because the critical issues that push them to move are not necessarily related to salary or benefits. Instead they are concerned about crime rates, the status of women, or family values. The level of crime in society cannot be underestimated as a reason to migrate. In South Africa more than 95 percent of emigrants cited high crime rates as their reason for emigrating.[20]

The *career-move migrant* is motivated by enhanced career opportunities either for herself or her family. The affirmative action policy recently introduced in South Africa indirectly limits career opportunities for white children and has encouraged the emigration of white families. This highlights the fact that political contexts and policies change over time and influence different groups of the population to migrate.

The *partner migrant* is another important category. Partner migration is particularly common among women, who often follow a husband or fiancé to another country. While they may be consulted before the move, they are not the principal interested party in this migration scenario.

The *adventurer migrant* is a smaller but no less important category. This adventurer uses nursing qualifications to finance travel to a destination country with no intention of returning to the source country in the immediate future. The main motivation is to have new experiences and visit exciting, unfamiliar places.

Using nursing to experience different cultures and see exotic sites may not be the primary motivation of most migrants, but it is often used as an added inducement to encourage nurses to migrate to nurse-starved locations. In the 1960s, for example, some recruiters offered migrating nurses from the Philippines stopovers in Tokyo and Hong Kong. Hospitals in the United States advertised the advantages of their cities—Chicago was portrayed as the nation's transportation hub—to recruit nurses keen to explore new vistas. Showing the Brooklyn Bridge and the Manhattan skyline, one recruitment firm claimed, "We will help you cross the BRIDGE from where you are to where you want to be."[21] These same inducements are alive and well today.

Survival migrants are motivated by goals that seem entirely opposite to those of adventurers. For them, life is far too much of an adventure already. Although they may not need to apply for political asylum, they are desperately trying to escape a situation of political oppression or armed conflict. Displaced persons or victims of natural disasters may also fall in this category. Their situation is often more critical than the level of need generally associated with the economic migrant.

And of course, there is the *return migrant,* someone who has worked for a period abroad and returns to the country of origin either temporarily or permanently. The reintegration of the return migrant poses, in many cases, quite unique and sometimes significant challenges.

Permanent migration is not the only kind that exists today. Many nurses, initially at least, consider themselves to be temporary migrants. Some, for example, are *holiday workers,* recent graduates or young professionals with some experience who want to acquire new knowledge and techniques while exploring unfamiliar cultures and broadening personal horizons. Solidly built into their travel plans is the intention of returning to the source country. This type of migration is so popular that many countries have specific work permits that facilitate entry of the holiday worker. Australia is a good example. Australia offers "working holiday visas" to young people (eighteen to thirty years old) of several European countries, including Italy, France, Cyprus, and the United Kingdom as well as countries in Asia like Japan, Hong Kong, and the Republic of Korea. Visa holders may remain in Australia for one year and obtain incidental work while traveling. These visas are awarded to thousands of workers a year. During 2001–2 nearly forty-one thousand working holiday visits were reported to have come from the United Kingdom alone.

A qualified nurse who wishes to visit innovative facilities or programs, in order to apply newly acquired knowledge and skills in the home country, may temporarily become a *study tour nurse.* Many national nurses' associations organize study tours for nurses coming from abroad. For example, a delegation from Japan visited the elderly care facilities in Denmark in order to learn from their innovative twenty-four-hour community approach to deliver services to a growing segment of the population.

One of the most important forms of temporary migration is student migration. The *student migrant* wishes to enter a formal nursing education program at a basic or higher level and generally intends to return to the source country. An important spin-off of student migration is occurring today as physicians who want to migrate to a different country turn to nursing in order to make the move. In some instances, physicians who have already migrated but are unable to practice medicine decide to become nurses. The arduous, costly, and time-consuming process of gaining medical credentials in a foreign country effectively prevents many migrant physicians from practicing medicine in their new homeland. They use their health care expertise to fast-track into a new career within a familiar work environment. Nursing is seen as "a sure ticket to a better-paying job and the shortest route to gain immigrant status."[22]

In the world of globalization, there is yet another interesting new category of temporary nurse migrant, the *contract worker*. From the outset, the contract worker understands that he or she will work for a short period of time (or repeated time-limited stretches) in the destination country in order to earn additional income, supplement pension funds or savings, or improve job prospects in the home country. The example of the "commuting" Jamaica nurse is typical of this category of worker.[23] This nurse either spends her vacation time and days off working in the United States or accepts long-weekend assignments that usually provide additional bonuses as well as the basic pay. According to Dennis Brown, the monthly salary earned by 70 percent of the Jamaican nurses working in the United States in the late 1990s ranged between $1,500 and $2,500. The US salary earned in one week represented the equivalent of four times what a counterpart in Jamaica earned in a month.[24] It is easy to understand the attraction of working even for short periods of time in the United States, once the qualification and work permit process becomes routine.

Interviewing nurses in the Caribbean, researchers found that many of them had worked in the United States repeatedly for various periods of time during their career. This work abroad was interspersed with time at home with their families, thus benefiting both worlds. Some migration can be extremely short term.

The worsening nursing shortage across the globe feeds this new phenomenon. New types of contract workers are being created to address the gaps in nursing personnel experienced in many countries. Teams of health professionals are organized to travel from one country to another to offer specific contracted services. For example, Netcare (the South African–based Network Healthcare Holdings Ltd.), a private company which started by operating four hospitals in South Africa and now owns and manages sixty-two, recently formed Netcare International. According to its home page, "Netcare International is dedicated to expanding the group's business internationally by sharing expertise and skill."[25] Determined to "become a global, integrated healthcare organization," Netcare signed a contract with the National Health Service in the United Kingdom to run treatment centers that specialize in cataract surgery. Nurses included in these teams work for periods of five weeks to six months in the United Kingdom, after which they return to work in South Africa.

With the available data it is difficult to determine if the majority of nurse migration is temporary or permanent. Looking at national nurse registers may give an indication but not a definitive answer. For example, nurses in the United Kingdom are required to renew their registration every three years. Less than half of non-EU foreign registrants in 1995 reregistered in 1998, and 85 percent of departures occurred within four years of entry to the United Kingdom.[26] This suggests that more than three-quarters of these foreign nurses registered in 1995 were no longer in active nursing practice in the United Kingdom four years later. Assuming that all these nurses actually went to the United Kingdom and continued to practice their profession, this would indicate that most migrants move on relatively quickly either to another destination country or back home.

It is often difficult to distinguish between the temporary and the permanent migrant. Clear distinctions are impossible when immigration policy definitions of *temporary* differ from country to country and range from three months to ten years. There is also a tendency for *temporary* to become *permanent* at any given point in time. Denise Duvoisin*, European born but brought up and educated in the United States, originally decided to return to Europe for a year of work experience after graduating from nursing school. That was thirty years ago, and despite opportunities to return to the United States, she is still working in Europe and has no intention of going back.

Some nurses find that conditions change and migration is no longer attractive. Margaret O'Brien* from Ireland accepted a six-month contract to work abroad. This contract has been renewed several times, and she is now entering her third year of employment. She discovered that exceeding an arbitrary limit—more than two years abroad—has suddenly revised her status at home. Because O'Brien has spent so much time working abroad, she is no longer eligible for special discounted rates on her mortgage in Ireland. At the same time, she has found that the process of getting her foreign car inspected and insured in Switzerland (which was not a problem for a short-term stay) is now becoming complicated with bureaucratic procedures that are very time consuming. Contact with former friends and professional networks is becoming more difficult because of the long separation, and she often feels isolated. What was bearable for the short term may become so burdensome that she may return home.

Some nurses envision a short-term move only to find that the political situation in the home country may radically change while they are away. A nurse from East Africa, Haile Kahsay*, went abroad to pursue his post-basic education. While he was away, a coup in his native country installed a dictatorial regime. Kahsay realized that he could not return home without serious consequences for himself and his family. He explored possibilities of migrating permanently to another country and was accepted. His intended short and temporary migration turned out to be permanent.

Pushing and Pulling

When nurse migration is discussed, economists and policy makers commonly talk about the *push* and *pull*. Although this is typical policy jargon, the concepts of push and pull describe the two fundamental sets of central and intertwined factors that drive migration. Pull factors are the conditions and circumstances in the destination country that attract and facilitate the movement of nurses toward that country. But since most people do not easily abandon family, friends, and communities, strong motivating forces must push nurses to forsake their country of origin. Push factors are thus the conditions or circumstances that encourage nurses to leave their country or location of work.

Push and pull factors often mirror each other. A nurse who has a relatively low salary will be pushed out of her country and pulled toward a country where there are relatively high salaries. Pull factors include things like high remuneration, job satisfaction, safe work environment, better-resourced health systems, or professional development opportunities. Political and economic stability, travel opportunities, and the chance to take part in humanitarian assistance would also draw, or pull, nurses to a particular location.

Active recruitment strategies of the destination country strengthen the pull. Facilitation with the emigration process, family support, educational/employment opportunities for family members, and family reunion programs—all are considered significant pull factors. As mentioned, the presence of family and friends and a large expatriate community or diaspora in the destination country is a key and powerful pull factor.[27] The data suggest, however, that no matter how strong the pull factors of the destination country, no significant migration takes place without substantial push factors in the source country. These could include poor quality of life, high crime, armed conflict, political repression, and lack of education/employment opportunities for children or other family members.

In the model presented by Ashnie Padarath and colleagues,[28] among the push factors specifically linked with the health system of the source country are poor remuneration and salaries, lack of job satisfaction, work-associated risks (such as exposure to HIV/AIDS without the proper protection equipment), lack of resources to work effectively, economic instability, high workloads, poor management and leadership, discrimination, corruption, professional isolation, lack of further education, and the absence of career development opportunities. When nurses have a professional degree, have obtained advanced skills or been certified in a nursing specialty (for example, oncology or critical care), and still cannot find employment, this is an obvious and extreme push factor.

While remuneration levels are often considered to be the most influential push and pull factors, there is no consensus on the relative weight each individual factor has in the decision making. The importance of each one may also differ for the same individual over time. For example, new graduates with their whole life in front of them may be more likely to move, while nurses close to retirement age may find moving too difficult or simply not cost-effective. Family situations also affect the decision to emigrate. Single nurses may have more freedom of choice. On the other hand, single mothers with heavier financial responsibilities may be under greater pressure to find a better-paying position, although this means facing the dilemma of financial survival or family cohesion. Nurses may be loath to leave their children behind. However, if a family member can take care of their children, the nurse may be more easily persuaded to emigrate.

Changes in the financial prospects or economic stability of the source country may also constitute serious push factors. High inflation, out-of-reach mortgages, unfavorable currency exchange rates, and chronic devaluation in purchasing power render already poor salaries even less attractive.

To understand the complex balance in the seesaw between push and pull, it is useful to look at examples of countries where nurses are pushed into migration and where they are pulled. The Philippines is perhaps the ultimate and certainly the most discussed example of how government policies, economic conditions, and family expectations combine to push nurses to migrate. In this example the pull factors, generated by health services in industrialized countries attempting to address their nursing shortages, are seen to be fully exploited by the government and business sectors of a developing country with a nurse surplus. Indeed, it is worth discussing the Philippine model in some detail because a number of other developing countries—St. Vincent, India, Indonesia, and Malaysia—are rapidly taking the same path.

The Philippines

The Philippine archipelago in Southeast Asia is slightly larger than Arizona, slightly smaller than Italy, and has a population of more than eighty-six million. There are two official languages in the Philippines, Filipino (based on Tagalog) and English. The literacy rate is very high with close to 96 percent of the population fifteen years and above able to read and write. Forty percent of the population, however, live below the poverty line, and the unemployment rate in 2003 was 11.4 percent. That same year, the Philippines had an external debt of $56.7 billion and its per capita gross domestic product was estimated at $4,600.[29]

There are several aspects of the Philippines that make it an ideal case study in nurse migration. One is its fertility rate, another its high rate of unemployment, but perhaps the most significant is its historical relationship to the United States and nursing. When countries have a high birth rate, they tend to produce more workers than can be easily absorbed by their national labor market, given the existing economic and political structures. Surplus labor then becomes an ideal commodity for export. In fact, approximately seven million Filipinos, or roughly 10 percent of the population, now live abroad and can be found worldwide. It is estimated that 2,300 persons are deployed overseas every day and the total mass of migrants send back $8 billion in savings every year.[30]

The Philippines, which were ceded by Spain to the United States in 1898 following the Spanish-American War, attained independence in 1946. In the first half of the twentieth century the Philippines and the United States forged close colonial relationships that continue to have a tremendous impact on present-day labor migration, including nurse migration.

One highly significant facet in the colonial relationship between the United States and the Philippines was the introduction and development of Western-style nursing in this Asian country. As Lavinia Dock, a US nurse and cofounder of the International Council of Nurses (ICN), wrote in 1912, "Nursing in the Philippines has a history on which we may look back with satisfaction, for, while carried on almost entirely by Americans in the early days of the occupation, its speedy adoption into the life and education of the Filipinos themselves and its wonderfully rapid development have probably not been surpassed elsewhere."[31] Could she have predicted that, by 1989, 73 percent of the foreign nurse graduates in the United States would be from the Philippines—with the second-largest group, Canadian nurses, falling far behind at 12 percent?[32]

According to Catherine Ceniza Choy's comprehensive history of Philippine nursing, the preconditions for this exodus began in 1907, when the US colonial government institutionalized nurse education. "From the beginning of U.S. colonial government-sponsored nursing training," Choy writes, "the study of English (grammar as well as colloquial English) was an integral part of the nursing students' curriculum."[33] Although other colonial governments, like the British in India, instituted training of health professionals, this important English-language component, missing in other developing countries, would prove crucial to Philippine migration. The education of nurses in the Philippines mirrored US patterns. Nurses constituted a predominantly female workforce recruited from socially respectable families and were sequestered in "the protected environment of the hospital."[34] Like American nursing students, Filipino students were all expected to share the same "work culture," living and working on the hospital grounds and providing a cheap or maybe free workforce for the hospital.

Nursing schools, important players in the migration of Filipino nurses, were established by a variety of entrepreneurial actors. For decades they have produced the steady supply of nurses needed to fill a fluctuating but nonetheless apparently enduring international demand. "The prestige and transformative potential of work abroad changed the culture of Philippine nursing training by encouraging not only thousands of other Filipino nurses to go to the United States, but also other young Filipino women to enter nursing school in the hopes of going abroad."[35] In the 1960s existing Filipino schools of nursing could not adequately supply the market, nor could they accommodate the increasing number of student applicants attracted by job offers abroad.

In 1966 the Philippine government deliberately encouraged entrepreneurial activity in the area of nursing education. The government passed an act that eased regulations on nursing schools in terms of maintaining hospital beds for clinical placements and providing an adequate library, classrooms, teaching equipment, and supplies. As a result, the establishment of a nursing school was less burdensome and thus even more attractive. Entrepreneurs in the Philippines thus accelerated the opening of schools in rural and urban areas. Their numbers grew from 17 to 140 between 1950 and 1970. "The increase in nursing schools continued," Choy writes, "because the owners of these schools earned huge profits from the tuition and other related expenses of their students."[36]

They still do. At the start of 2005, there were some 370 nursing programs operating in the country.[37] Many worry that the government regulatory body cannot adequately monitor the schools and enforce the minimum education standards. Lowering the knowledge and skill level of new graduates affects the marketability of the final product, a direct financial threat to the multitude now involved in the recruitment chain. The greater risk, however, is to the students who have invested in a university education that may not hold its promise of providing the knowledge and skills that will allow them to pass their qualifying or licensing exams.

Choy argues that "the U.S. introduction of professional nursing greatly influenced Filipino women in ways that were both liberating and exploitative."[38] The fact remains that nursing education in the early 1900s provided a range of prestigious professional opportunities that had not existed under the previous Spanish reign. The demand for nurses not only continues to support an expanding private education industry but also provides a labor export for the country and a sure pass into the international labor market. It has reached the point now that an increasing number of Filipino physicians (two thousand in 2001 and twice as many in 2004) are switching to the nursing profession in order to board the "gravy train" of international nurse recruitment. This professional recycling is not limited to physicians. In 2004 numerous Filipino engineers and lawyers—and even one fifty-five-year-old judge—took the nursing licensure exam in order to obtain employment in the United States and thus improve their earning power and pension benefits.[39]

Since 1948, when the United States established the Exchange Visitor Program (and its various successors), the government facilitated the entry of Filipino nurses. Government, employers, recruitment agencies, travel agencies, educational institutions—all saw the value of encouraging Filipino nurses to migrate. Hospital employers began to initiate orientation programs tailored to the Filipino nurse. Even the American Nurses Association actively campaigned. In 1962 it sent out a brochure titled "Your Cap Is Your Passport" to nursing organizations across the globe, including the Philippines.[40]

The flow of nurses began in earnest, and an estimated twenty-five thousand Filipino nurses emigrated to the United States between 1966 and 1985. In the 1970s some Filipino leaders expressed concern about the mass exodus of nurses, but many others defended the nurses' choice to emigrate. One nurse educator, Conchita B. Ruiz, urged other Filipinos to consider the high unemployment in the Philippines, the low wages of government employees, and the poor working conditions and inadequate facilities.[41]

The situation remains essentially unchanged today. The Philippine government continues to actively support nurse emigration in order to ease the heavy burden of unemployment at home and encourage the transfer of hard currency remittances (individual savings sent to families back home) that will improve the population's financial viability and survival. For 2004 alone, the Bangko Sentral ng Pilipinas received US$8.5 billion—nearly 10 percent of the country's gross national product, more than half of the 2005 national budget.

Reports of nursing shortages in the Philippines are starting once again to be heard. In the very same articles, however, are quotes from dueling experts who contradict one another. In a recent reported interview, Dr. Jaime Galvez Tan, vice-chancellor for research at the University of the Philippines in Manila, voices alarm because there are no nurses in large areas of Mindanao (a site of continual armed conflict and social unrest) and that the nurse-to-patient ratio in Manila instead of being 1:20 is now 1:40 or in some cases 1:60. Yet Rosalinda Baldoz, administrator of the Philippines Overseas Employment Administration, quoted in the same article, admits, "When you look at reality here, the (nurses') salary is low. Graduates can't find work so there are limited options, like applying for jobs that do not match their skills or settling for low paychecks."[42]

Diego Bañez*, like many nurses in the Philippines, entered the profession for the opportunity to travel overseas to work. After graduation Bañez was unable to find paid employment in the Philippines. His only option was volunteer work in a hospital. During his first two years of clinical experience in the operating theaters of a private hospital, he survived on the allowances given to him by visiting surgeons. Dissatisfied with this impossible situation, he emigrated to New Zealand and is now working in Australia.[43] His is not an isolated example. In spite of the concern over the imminent shortage of skilled nurses and the high vacancy rates in rural areas, many newly educated nurses in the Philippines are unable to find a good job. To keep up their skills and gain the clinical experience necessary for employment, many nurses are obliged to work in hospitals for nothing.[44] In fact, because foreign health employers are increasingly targeting nurses with some working experience, such voluntary servitude becomes critical to migration. Highly exploitative conditions are thus created and make migration the only viable professional option. Similar situations have been reported in various African countries, for example, Tanzania and Zambia, as well as in Eastern Europe.

Developing Countries

Emigration from the Philippines began far earlier than in most developing countries. The massive migration now seen in other countries mirrors some of the Philippine experience. But global nurse migration has been significantly enhanced—pushed—by recent economic policies (paradoxically called public-sector reform or health system restructuring) that have depleted health system budgets and made the creation of satisfying nursing careers in developing countries an uphill battle and at times virtually a mission impossible.

In Africa, as in many developing countries, the public-sector "reform" process, which started in the mid-1980s, was executed through structural adjustment programs of the World Bank and the International Monetary Fund calling for downsizing or zero growth in the public sector. For over two decades, the IMF prescription for troubled third world economies remained consistent. The basic principles are neatly summarized by Robin Hanhel in his book *Panic Rules!*[45]

The first step is monetary austerity—tightening up the money supply to increase internal interest rates to whatever heights are needed to stabilize the value of the local currency. Next comes fiscal austerity—increasing tax collections and dramatically reducing government spending. The third step is privatization—selling off public enterprises to the private sector. And finally, financial liberalization—removing restrictions on the inflow and outflow of international capital as well as restrictions on what foreign businesses and banks are allowed to buy, own, and operate. Once governments accept these conditions, the IMF agrees to lend the countries enough money to prevent default on international loans about to come due (thus avoiding bankruptcy). It also then arranges a restructuring of the country's debt among private international lenders, imposing a pledge of new loans.

According to Ann-Louise Colgan, writing in *Africa Action*, "the past two decades of World Bank and IMF structural adjustment in Africa have led to greater social and economic deprivation, and an increased dependence of African countries on external loans. The failure of structural adjustment has been so dramatic that some critics of the World Bank and IMF argue that the policies imposed on African countries were never intended to promote development."[46] Colgan goes on to say that these policies have caused a deterioration in health and in health care services across the African continent.

The IMF policies have had a direct impact on the health sector and its personnel in multiple ways. Monetary austerity increased the cost of everything, including mortgage rates and food. Since salaries tend not to rise in these situations, workers' real income automatically decreased, buying less with the same amount of money. Reducing government spending led to health-sector budget cuts, which in turn resulted in a general downsizing of health facilities. A reduction in the number of financed positions in the public sector, the largest employer in most developing countries, can only lead to widespread unemployment unless provisions for alternative work are made. The hope was that a budding private sector could absorb these workers. This proved to be an illusion.

For those remaining in the public sector, workloads dramatically increased, working conditions eroded, and the level of stress nurses experienced escalated. Finally, privatizing the public sector often resulted in increasing the price of vital daily commodities and services—water, fuel, gas, electricity, health care. Health care administrators and employers in the private sector tended to renegotiate workers' contracts, usually offering workers lower salaries, less benefits, and no job security.

At the turn of this century, World Bank and IMF evaluations of structural adjustment programs initiated in the 1980s revealed the devastation they had left behind. To give but one example, measures affecting the health sector in Cameroon "resulted in suspending recruitment, strict implementation of retirement at 50 or 55, limiting employment to 30 years, suspension of any financial promotion, reduction of additional benefits and two salary reductions—totaling 50% and a currency devaluation resulting in an effective income loss of 70% over 15 years. In addition, paramedical training for nurses and laboratory technicians was suspended for several years and schools closed. . . . In 1999, jobs in the public sector were about 80% unfilled, and Cameroon had a truly de-motivated health workforce."[47]

Early retirement packages or "golden handshakes" were increasingly introduced, even in countries like South Africa. New graduates started having difficulty finding jobs. Despite research demonstrating their cost-effectiveness in the delivery of a wide range of health services, nurses looking for employment were turned away. The important role of nurses in meeting the increasing health needs of a growing population was minimized or ignored. Large numbers of nurses became part of the unemployed, including in Africa where the needs continued to be enormous.[48]

The impact of reform as an important migration push factor in the health-sector workforce was the focus of a World Bank background paper on the human resource crisis in health services in sub-Saharan Africa. The paper describes the havoc found today. "Results of these [restructuring] measures on . . . health personnel were not dramatically different from one country to another. The impact is a lasting one, largely determining the attitudes of health providers and the actual availability of health personnel. . . . Although availability of health personnel is a critical issue, a review of World Bank documents in six African countries found that this issue was not adequately taken into consideration—either in magnitude or in dimension. Moreover, health workforce issues were often not considered . . . preventing governments from addressing workforce shortages."[49]

Given this history, one might think that health planners would place a high priority on workforce issues. Unfortunately, the WHO observes that "workforce issues are still considered to be relatively unimportant by both national governments and international agencies [although] limitations on staffing are now recognized as a major constraint to achieving national health goals."[50] For example, the government in Mali aggressively increased the number of community health posts to 533 to meet health needs of the population in rural areas. However, only 43 percent of them were operational in January 2001, the others having been closed down for lack of personnel.[51]

Attracting and retaining health professionals in rural areas is particularly difficult. Looking at workforce data from Ghana, Guinea, and Senegal, more than 50 percent of the nurses are concentrated in the capital city, where less than 20 percent of the population lives.[52] In an effort to remedy this maldistribution of personnel, countries like South Africa have put in place special allowances to recruit more professionals to areas away from the capital city, and as compensation for the additional hardships often encountered in rural postings. While these inducements may work to a certain degree, the wrong message is sent when the percentages of salary allocated to the different disciplines varies.

In South Africa the minister of health, Dr. Manto Tshabalala-Msimang, announced the introduction in 2004 of rural allowances which apply to thirty-three thousand health professionals, including professional nurses, working in designated areas.[53] The proposal to grant allowances resulting in wage increases of 22 percent to physicians but only 12 percent to nurses was regarded as an insult to the nursing profession.[54] With the wage disparities already present, a difference in allocation percentage sends an unacceptable blow to nurses and tangible proof of the lower value placed on their skills. A similar situation exists with South Africa's scarce skills allowance. The proposed percentage of salary increase allocated to physicians is 18 percent while nurses received only 8 percent. The nurses' national professional union, DENOSA, responded immediately, advocating common allowance rates. The organization argued that when remuneration rates are so low, compared to physician compensation, this sends a negative message that will discourage new recruits to nursing.

Both in the developing world and in industrialized countries, the workforce has rarely been a priority. "Workforce issues are still nowhere near the top of the agenda for [UK] managers or trust boards, who have other managerial 'must dos,' such as reducing waiting lists and times, managing emergency admissions, and breaking even financially."[55] The link between adequate staffing and achieving health targets goes largely unnoticed and unheeded.

It seems, however, that the international community has now recognized the devastating impact previous policies have had on health care. In 2000 the 189 United Nations member states endorsed the Millennium Development Goals. This unprecedented agreement by the development community focuses energy and resources on the attainment of eight goals, eighteen targets, and forty-eight performance indicators relating to poverty reduction by 2015. Application of the approved strategies will necessarily be international in scope and labor intensive. Since health is both negatively affected by poverty and at the same time constitutes an essential resource for self-sufficiency and productivity, the health sector has an important role to play in the realization of these goals. A search for personnel to initiate the MDG programs quickly revealed the desperate situation most developing countries face, given their seriously depleted public sectors. Consequently, the majority of funds raised to achieve the Millennium Development Goals will have to be spent on building effective workforces that will deliver essential services to the population.[56] Pushing aside the substantial downsizing exercise of past years, the international community is now looking for ways to increase the supply of nurses in developing countries. Only time will tell if their efforts in rebuilding the nursing workforce will be as successful as they were in depleting it.

It is clear that during the 1990s reform in the developing countries significantly downsized the health care workforce in general and nursing in particular. In many countries this set the stage for mass nurse migration. But, as has been mentioned, economic reform could not have pushed so many nurses out of developing countries if accompanying pull factors in the industrialized world did not create a hospitable environment for foreign recruits.

Interestingly, similar hospital restructuring policies had been introduced in the industrialized countries, thus greatly downsizing their nursing workforce in the late 1980s and early 1990s. As in the developing countries, nurses were pushed out of jobs and often unemployed. Nursing became a lost paradise for those nurses who remained in health care and had to cope with greatly increased workloads, stress, and job dissatisfaction. Reduced student pools, high turnover rates, low job satisfaction, and increased opportunities of employment outside the health sector resulted in a decreased number of nurses willing to work in the health services of industrialized countries. This in turn dramatically affected the wider international labor market. In the late 1990s, faced with a sudden increased demand for health services by an aging population and expanded community services, health-sector employers turned to foreign workers to fill nursing vacancies. The critical shortage of nurses in the industrialized countries thus became a major pull factor that to a great extent explains the vacuum effect and aggressive international recruitment practiced since the mid-1990s.

The Nursing Shortage—the New Pull

It is now commonplace to hear about catastrophic worldwide nursing shortages. This concept of shortage is, however, worth briefly exploring. A shortage implies a comparison between current conditions and a calculated and desired norm. That norm may be defined in the context of demand or need. *Demand* is an economic term. It is the amount of a service (in this case nursing care) that consumers—employers or clients—would be willing to acquire at a given price. *Need,* on the other hand, is a subjective judgment about the ideal amount of a product or service that should be available regardless of the price. The person who directly pays for the product or service usually decides demand. Need in the health sector is most often determined by professional associations or health planners.

This distinction is crucial. When considering the number of nurses in a given country, area, or facility, it is possible for those who finance health care—whether they be governments, private employers, or insurance companies—to insist that there is no shortage in terms of demand, whereas in fact there is a shortage when one considers need. In other words, all budgeted nursing positions may be filled, but the number of nurses a government or health facility is willing to allot simply cannot deal with the level of patient need, generating gaps in services.

In Spain, for example, an estimated thirteen thousand unemployed nurses are being aggressively recruited by France, Portugal, Italy, the United Kingdom, and other countries. The professional associations in Spain are concerned. They argue that, when it comes to nursing, the Spanish people are receiving inadequate health service coverage. These associations are actively lobbying for an additional one hundred thousand nurse positions in order to meet national health needs. While demand-oriented payers may insist that the health system has a nursing surplus, need-focused organizations will argue that there is a shortage. Unfortunately, the balance between need and demand is rarely attained, and in today's cost-conscious climate, planners, researchers, and writers tend to use demand as the basis for analysis and calculation.[57] Too often, patient need takes second place to financial considerations.

The severity and breadth of the present shortage, which really began in the late 1990s, has attracted serious attention and fueled many discussions. Since World War II, the cyclical nature of nurse shortages and surpluses in the industrialized countries often encouraged policy makers to take a laissez-faire attitude. In the United States, for example, market forces were allowed to exercise their power freely in an environment where little external competition for nurse employment was exerted by other sectors. Until recently, "hospitals tended not to compete with one another for nurses. . . . Nurses' real wages show sustained periods of stagnation culminating in increased hospital nurse vacancy rates generally followed by an industry-wide wage response and vacancy reductions. The cyclical pattern repeats itself about every 7 years."[58] In countries where the public sector dominated the provision of health services, similar although perhaps more subtle market forces and cyclical shortages were present.

Although the health sector expanded in the 1970s and 1980s in both the industrialized countries and the developing world,[59] health-sector work-forces began to be seriously reduced globally in the mid-1980s to 1990s when economic downturns and changes in the financing systems of health services imposed dramatic budget cuts. The health workforce was seen as a drain on the budget rather than an essential resource to be fully utilized for social development or marketed for financial gain. As mentioned, important cost-cutting measures were implemeited and, in many countries, the nursing workforce was the major target.[60]

Nurses are the largest category of health care professionals, and their salaries represent the biggest single expenditure item for hospitals (approximately 20 percent).[61] In the industrialized countries, cost-cutting and cost-containment measures began to change the shape of the health sector as well as its practices. Restructuring has meant "increased emphasis on private enterprise; changes in payment systems; shortened hospital stays; higher proportions of acute care patients; expansion of community-based services, including home-care; and greater emphasis on cost control."[62] Waves of redundancy became commonplace.

Nurses looking for employment were sent away while cheaper substitutes, care assistants with little education or training, often replaced them. The use of part-time employment and temporary work increased, contributing to a sense of job insecurity that was new to the nursing profession. Nurses began exploring other sectors for alternative career opportunities. Abandoning their profession became some nurses' only viable solution.

Push factors clearly contributed to the decrease in homegrown nurses' willingness to work and the desperate need of health-sector employers to create attractive pull factors that might seduce migrant nurses to fill the perpetually created vacancies. The United States, often at the forefront of change, is a good example.

The United States

The United States, with its population of more than 293 million, is said to have the largest and most technologically powerful economy in the world with a per capita gross domestic product of $37,800.[63] There are 2.7 million registered nurses licensed to practice, of which 500,000 choose not to work in nursing or are unemployed. To meet its health system demand, the United States must recruit one million nurses into active practice before 2010.

In the United States almost 60 percent of all hospitals undertook restructuring initiatives during 1991–96. Of these, personnel were reduced in roughly 90 percent; registered nurses were laid off in 25 percent, and nearly 50 percent lost registered nurses through voluntary resignations as a result of substantial nurse dissatisfaction.[64] In fact, job dissatisfaction among US hospital nurses is four times greater than the average for all workers in the country.[65] Nurses insist that heavy workloads—working with too many patients with intense needs—prevent them from giving quality care. They are frustrated by the inadequate resources, insufficient time for patients, weak staff support, and lack of voice in the decision-making process. Nurses tend to be given responsibility and be held accountable for patient care, even though they have little or no authority to control their work environment or workplace policies. Linda Aiken, a nursing workforce researcher, insists that "nurse burnout is driven less by the stresses inherent in caring for very ill people and more by organizational impediments to the delivery of an acceptable standard of nursing care, especially inadequate resources and poor administrative support."[66]

During recent decades the population growth in industrialized countries has for the most part slowed, ceased, or even reversed.[67] The population is going gray—getting older, sometimes much older. Low birth rates and an increased life expectancy are transforming national demographic profiles. It is also having a direct impact on the tax revenue available to support public health systems, since income taxes collected from a shrinking pool of productive workers have to fund medical care for a growing number of older people.

While it is difficult to accurately predict consumer demand or patient need, the increasing population of older persons certainly plays a dominant role in determining the quantity as well as type of services and personnel required in the coming years. Already in the United States, 48 percent of total 1999 hospital inpatient days and 40 percent of all short-stay hospital discharges are linked to care of persons sixty-five years or older.[68] Governments and employers must adjust their budgets to finance the posts required to meet the needs of older persons in various settings—hospitals, rehabilitation centers, home care, day care centers, and residential homes. The number of nursing homes has also greatly increased in recent years, thus expanding the labor market and increasing the demand for nurses, often met by migrant professionals.

Yet, the restructuring of the late 1980s and early 1990s downsized not only health care facilities but also educational institutions. The number of nursing schools and nursing student positions fell. Mistaken forecasting compounded the situation. In the United States, a prediction in 1995 of an oversupply of nurses by 200,000 to 300,000 by the end of the twentieth century led to a recommendation for closure of 10 to 25 percent of nursing schools.[69] As a consequence, the subsequent cohorts of nursing students were dramatically reduced in size, a fact that has contributed to the inadequate supply of nurses today.

In parallel, new health-sector financing systems such as *diagnosis-related groups* and *managed care* have been introduced in order to reduce the constantly rising health costs. Diagnosis-related groups are a mode of hospital financing whereby government or insurance companies pay a standard preestablished price for treatment of any given disease or surgical intervention. Hospitals then have a financial incentive to reduce patients' stay to the minimum extent possible. Managed care works on a similar basis. It is a system of health insurance characterized by a network of contracted providers, for example, health maintenance organizations (HMOs), that delivers health services to a defined population for a fixed payment. Again, built into the system is a financial incentive for whatever group of health professionals is involved—be they physicians or nurse practitioners or the HMOs themselves—to provide care at the lowest possible price.

Financing mechanisms seeking to minimize health care costs have influenced health systems in many countries. They have been a major force in shortening hospital stays, expanding outpatient departments (for example, day surgery), and encouraging general practice or community care. Cost-containment measures have increased the percentage of acute care patients in any given hospital unit. These services are generally under the responsibility of highly educated health care workers, namely, professional nurses. As patient acuity (illness severity) increases, so should the number of qualified nurses within the health care team. At the same time, the role of community nurses has expanded. They now have to deal with patients who have been discharged from hospital quickly and are therefore fragile and dependent on skilled care. Nurse practitioners, who tend to receive lower salaries than physicians yet provide a range of similar services—for example, care of the chronically ill—are considered increasingly attractive options in the delivery of quality care. This creates additional career opportunities for nurses, and at the same time the attraction of these new and better-paid jobs draws nurses away from work in bedside care.

Increasingly heavy workloads are a direct consequence of two intersecting phenomena. Hospitals have reduced the number of qualified nurses, and, because of the dramatically shortened length of hospital stay, these nurses are caring for patients with higher acuity. Thus, for example, a nurse will be caring for a greater number of patients who, because they are admitted for shorter amounts of time, have more intense needs. All of this not only has increased the risk to patients but has exacerbated occupational health hazards routinely present in the nurse workplace.

According to the US Joint Commission on Accreditation of Healthcare Organizations:

> Nurses have been described as the "canaries in the coal mine." Many have been sacrificed before the now widespread realization that there is something wrong with the work environment. Nurses leave hospitals because they are overworked and overburdened, often with tasks that were once the responsibilities of less skilled workers. They similarly have neither the managerial support nor the control over their environments—through delegated authority—to marshal and deploy scarce resources in order to manage the often challenging, and sometimes critical patient care situation which they may face at any hour of the day or night.[70]

The combination of biological, physical, chemical, social, and sensory health hazards has won nursing the dubious distinction of being one of the most dangerous professions today. According to a study done by the American Nurses Association, 75 percent of nurses surveyed stated that unsafe working conditions interfere with their ability to provide quality care. Nearly 90 percent of the respondents claim that health and safety concerns influence the type of nursing work they do and the likelihood of their remaining in active practice.[71]

Given this context, it is hardly a shock that relatively smaller numbers of students are willing to enter nursing. The percentage of registered nurses under the age of thirty decreased by 41 percent, while in the general US workforce the percentage fell only 1 percent between 1983 and 1998.[72] This suggests that the share of young people entering nursing is decreasing. In fact, women graduating from high school in the late 1980s and 1990s were 35 percent less likely to choose nursing as a career than women graduating from high school in the 1970s.[73]

According to the Royal College of Nursing of the United Kingdom, "Historically nursing has sometimes been regarded as a low-status profession due to the low levels of pay and heavy workloads. This makes the individuals doing the job appear all the more valuable."[74] Hence an apparent paradox: nurses, as individuals, are highly regarded, but the work that they do, nursing, often is not.

While the average age of nurses in developing countries continues to be in the early to mid thirties, nurses from industrialized countries tend to be ten years older. For example, the average age of nurses in the United States and Sweden is forty-five, in Canada forty-four, and in New Zealand and Denmark forty-three.[75] The rate of average age increase is also of interest; in the United States, nursing is aging more than twice as fast as all other occupations.[76] In concrete terms, approximately 50 percent of the nursing workforce is forty-five years of age or older and is expected to retire in the next ten to fifteen years.[77] The average age of United States nursing faculty is even higher: fifty. The threat that retirement will rapidly reduce the already depleted numbers of nurse educators is a very real one. It brings with it serious implications for future generations of nursing students, who will increasingly find entry to education programs difficult, followed by bottlenecks in their training due to the absence of clinical instructors.

Interestingly, there has been a noted increase in the number of mature students in nursing education programs. This has happily filled the gap left by the shrinking pool of high school graduates. The professional life of a mature student is generally shorter, however, because of the reduced numbers of years between qualifying and retirement.

The American Hospital Association reports that there are currently 126,000 nurse vacancies in US hospitals and that if nothing is done, these vacancies will increase to 400,000 by 2006. As mentioned, it is estimated that the United States must recruit one million nurses by 2010 to cover nursing needs in hospitals, community care, schools, rehabilitation centers, and nursing homes.

The demand for health services is very sensitive to fluctuations in the economy. With the recent slight improvement of the US economy since 2000, the demand for health services suddenly increased. The health sector is presently one of the principal growth industries, and the US Bureau of Labor Statistics ranks the occupation of nursing as having the seventh-highest projected job growth in the country.[78] According to Reed Abelson,

After years in which they closed beds and laid off workers, many hospitals are struggling to cope with surprising increases in the number of patients. . . . Hospital admissions are hovering at levels last seen in the mid-1980s. Just over 33 million people were admitted to hospitals in 2000, the latest year for which statistics are available. . . . That was up from a low of 30.7 million in 1994. Outpatient visits have also increased, climbing 16%, to 521 million, since 1997. . . . A 2002 industry study [issued by the Society for Healthcare Strategy and Market Development] concluded, "After 10 years of downsizing in the 1990s, hospitals are making new building plans."[79]

John Rivers, president of the Arizona Hospital and Healthcare Association, observes that almost every hospital in the state has completed their plans or has plans under way to increase their capacity. Although hospital strategic development departments now focus on expansion, their progress is blocked because of the key issue of nurse shortages.[80]

Other Examples

The situation in other industrialized countries is very similar. Fifty percent of nurses employed in Canada today will retire within the next fifteen years. In order to replace the huge cohorts of the 1970s, graduate levels of four to five thousand per year will be required just to maintain actual levels of the nurse workforce. However, the estimated *increase* in demand for nursing services in Canada is 53 percent by the year 2015. In order for the nurse workforce to expand sufficiently, student numbers should not only be maintained but substantially increase.[81] In fact, graduating classes in recent years have shrunk by one or two thousand students nationwide, thus exacerbating the decrease in supply. There are plans to increase the output from Canada's nursing schools to more than nine thousand per annum by the year 2007. Projections, however, suggest that there will still be a nurse shortfall of 331,000 in 2011 and 361,000 in 2016.[82]

There is no doubt that labor needs exist and are exerting rising pressure on health authorities and private-sector health employers to find nurses to fill the empty slots. The United Kingdom needs to recruit eighty thousand nurses by 2008, while Australia will have an estimated shortfall of thirty-one thousand nurses by 2006. A recent snapshot survey commissioned by the Royal College of Nursing (UK) indicates widespread staff shortages. Eight in ten hospital wards reported that nurse staffing is inadequate and should be increased by 17 percent. When replacements for nurses on maternity leave or long-term sick leave are added to the picture, staff is functioning at a level 13 percent below optimal.[83] The nursing workforce specialist Keith Hurst recently described the situation in the United Kingdom: "Direct patient care is falling by about 1% every year. It used to be that nurses spent 70% of their time in face-to-face contact with patients. This is now down to about 48%."[84]

Occupational Health Hazards and Nurse Supply

Nurses are prime targets for physical and psychological workplace violence. When the Joint Programme on Workplace Violence of the ILO, ICN, WHO, and Public Services International (PSI) studied the problem, they found that workplace violence is pervasive and widespread. Verbal abuse, bullying, and sexual harassment were among the most common forms of violence; these incidents were found to be as traumatic as physical assault.[85] While patients and their families tend to be the perpetrators of physical violence in the health-sector workplace, colleagues and supervisors are most often responsible for the unacceptably high rate of psychological violence. More than half of the responding health personnel had experienced at least one incident of physical or psychological violence in the year previous to the Joint Programme study: 76 percent in Bulgaria, 67 percent in Australia, 61 percent in South Africa, 54 percent in Thailand, and 47 percent in Brazil. Ambulance staff, nurses, and doctors reported suffering the highest offense rates. Recognition of workplace violence as an important generator of post-traumatic stress disorders (PTSD) is an uncontroversial major finding of all the country surveys. Between 40 and 70 percent of victims reported significant levels of PTSD symptoms.[86] The correlation between violence and stress is of particular significance in the light of the high levels of stress reported worldwide within health care settings.

Indeed, workplace violence is so toxic that nurses increasingly report that it is one reason they abandon active practice. Aiken refers to the increase in violence by patients and their families in health care settings as a type of "ward rage" stimulated by a general sense of frustration and dissatisfaction with the quality of care received. This behavior compromises the civility of the work environment and contributes to the high rates of nurse burnout.[87]

Physicians' disrespect and abuse are also serious problems, and Suzanne Gordon details some of the many situations nurses face when physicians do not understand their work or are verbally or physically abusive.[88] Similarly, Diana Mason, editor of the *American Journal of Nursing*, recalls a situation where "in one hospital, nurses, administrators, and other physicians did nothing about a surgeon who had tantrums if the operating room temperature wasn't just right (he actually threw instruments at nurses). The nursing director dismissed it as 'stress.' It was an environment I couldn't stay in for long."[89] Many nurses agree. In a survey of twelve hundred nurses and other hospital staff published in the *American Journal of Nursing*, nearly one-third said they knew of a nurse who had left a job because of physician abuse.[90]

Maggie Marum, a former primary care director, interviewed nurses and general practitioners who had left the British National Health Service. Almost half of the nurses cited the bullying, inflexible, or hierarchical management as the reason for their abandoning employment. Says one nurse, "When I go to work I expect to be treated as a human being, but there are a lot of bullies in nurse management. The managers were very unsupportive and undermined experienced nurses' confidence."[91] While the sample of this particular study was very small, it confirmed the findings of larger studies that report a wide prevalence of psychological abuse in the health sector.

Sick leave and lowered productivity are often side effects of occupational accidents and diseases. "Nurses greatly stressed and vulnerable to injury have a higher absentee and disability rate than almost any other profession, which disrupts care, makes planning difficult and costs the health care system a great deal of money."[92] Not only does the concern for personal safety dissuade people from entering or remaining in the nursing profession, it also has consequences in terms of temporary absence from the workplace. This increases the workload of colleagues and has a negative impact on the quality of care. Dealing with the increasing number of occupational accidents and diseases is also costly, diverting necessary funds from employing and retaining nurses in sufficient numbers.

Pay and Supply

While working conditions were mentioned most frequently as the reason nurses leave active practice, pay came in second. Once a living wage is reached, nurses tend to be more concerned about the relatively unfavorable salaries they receive.[93] The substantial wage disparities commonly found between nurses and other workers, even when they are professionals possessing comparable educational requirements and holding similar degrees of responsibility, are felt to be denigrating and a major source of frustration. The Royal College of Nursing estimates that a pay raise of 20 percent for nurses would be needed if equally qualified nurses and police constables were to have comparable salaries.[94] Laila Harré from the New Zealand Nurses Organization observes that "in comparison with similar groups, including police, teachers and other health professionals, our research shows nurses and midwives are paid between $7,000 and $15,000 a year less than they are worth."[95] Incomes of teachers in the most recent British household panel survey averaged 50 percent higher than nurses. Such dramatic increases in salary are unlikely anytime soon. Wage disparities will continue to cast a shadow on the profession. The relative income of nurses within their home countries is a critical influence on attrition and migration.[96]

Research on job satisfaction demonstrates that if working conditions are satisfactory and relationships between colleagues in the workplace are positive, the importance of salary diminishes.[97] Even when working conditions and collegial relationships are good, nurses are still dismayed when they read the newspapers and find that hospital maintenance workers or toilet cleaners are paid the same or higher salaries than qualified nurses. In 1987 hospital maintenance workers in the Washington DC area earned $25,000 per year whereas the average hospital staff nurse salary was $23,753.[98] A more recent example shows that the practice continues. In Guildford, England, toilet cleaners were offered a salary of £12,480 in 1998 while registered nurses (D-grade) earned just £400 a year more.[99]

The different treatment given to male-dominated versus female-dominated professions is found in developing countries. A pay-equity exercise undertaken in the Philippines found that a carpenter foreman earns a salary of ₱8,709. His responsibilities include supervising carpentry work, scheduling job orders, and preparing cost estimates. Experience and technical training are the only qualifications for this job. Midwives, on the other hand, require tertiary-level midwifery education and licensure. They give prenatal and post-delivery care to women, deliver babies, chart the newborn's and mother's health, and instruct student midwives—all for a salary of ₱7,606.

Now that women have more career options than they had in the past, such salary differentials make it difficult to recruit to the profession. Whereas previous generations of women were frequently restricted to nursing, teaching, and administrative work, current generations can choose from a wide selection of careers, including engineering, law, banking, and medicine. Nursing, as a predominately female profession, has greatly suffered from gender discrimination and is often less well paid than typically male-dominated professions. Even when nurses enjoy similar levels of starting pay, other disciplines tend to offer better long-term pay, more promotional opportunities, family-friendly hours, a safer work environment, and more prestige.

It is not surprising that people outside the profession are hesitant to enter nursing when an increasing percentage of nurses feel they cannot recommend nursing as a career. In a recent survey undertaken by the American Nurses Association, nearly 55 percent of participating nurses would not recommend nursing to their children or friends and 23 percent of the respondents would actively discourage someone from entering the profession.[100]

In the United Kingdom, this figure was even higher. The Royal College of Nursing found that 62 percent of responding nurses would not recommend nursing as a career.[101] This high level of dissatisfaction and frustration is bound to communicate itself to others.

Statistics released by the Australian Institute of Health and Welfare paint an equally pessimistic picture. There is a "decline in new entrants in nursing—with students completing nursing courses falling by 20% between 1993 and 2000 and the number commencing falling by 4% between 1999 and 2000."[102] The insufficient supply of student positions is alarming. Although the 2003 federal budget announced two hundred additional places in undergraduate nursing courses, a shortfall of thirty-one thousand was expected by 2006. Approximately three thousand eligible applicants were refused in 2003, however, due to the lack of university places and clinical placements.

In the United Kingdom, the total number of nursing and midwifery students has almost doubled between 1995 and 2000. But this increase may do little more than compensate for cuts in education imposed in the 1980s and early 1990s.[103] Of these students, one in every five in England and Wales, and one in every four in Scotland and Northern Ireland, abandons the nursing program before completion.[104] The greatest shock comes with the realization that among the new graduates, those that actually finish the study program, one-third never register to practice.[105] In all likelihood, they are completely lost to the profession. In New Zealand, only 60 percent of graduates who register remain active in the workforce after three years, with the proportion dropping to 48 percent after nine to eleven years.[106] Similarly, evidence gathered in Ireland suggest that up to 70 percent of newly qualified Irish nurses have left the national health service within eighteen months of graduation.[107]

Shortage: Myth or Reality?

Any attempts to regulate the workforce environment and avoid periodic shortages or surpluses have tended to be cosmetic and short-term. In the light of the widespread, urgent, and increasing need and demand for nurses, this type of approach can no longer be justified. The absence of well-founded human resources planning and management is evident and repeatedly blamed for the current crisis situation.[108] Despite a growing supply of registered nurses in absolute numbers, the lack of nurses has had a dramatic impact on patients and health care systems as well as economic and social development. Intolerably high nurse vacancy rates are no longer the lot of developing countries alone. With few exceptions, nursing shortages are a priority concern everywhere. Predictions that this situation will continue for at least ten to twenty years are alarming. Nurses have become very rare resources in an increasingly competitive global labor market.

Staggering figures are trumpeted to describe the massive shortage worldwide and project the negative impact it will have on patients as well as personnel. Yet, a few observers quietly suggest that this may all be a myth or a red herring. The lack of reliable data from many countries makes it difficult to resolve the question. What is certain is that in many countries there is a substantial national pool of licensed nurses who refuse to practice their profession. As reported, there are approximately half a million nurses in the United States—20 percent of all registered nurses—who renew their licenses to remain on the register but choose not to work in nursing under current conditions. There are many examples to indicate that nurses love their profession but hate the job.

According to the Joint Commission on the Accreditation of Healthcare Organizations, "overwhelmingly, nurses report that the most enjoyable aspect of being a nurse is helping patients and their families. The majority of nurses (74%) said they would stay at their jobs if changes were made. Top among the identified desirable changes were increased staffing, less paperwork, and fewer administrative duties."[109] Time will tell if policy makers and health-sector administrators will heed the call. Thus far, there is little cause for optimism.

The challenge of ensuring sufficient numbers of nurses in health services will only be met when serious attention is focused on retention issues—on increasing pay and making concrete and long-term changes in working conditions. Until then, retention problems will continue to sabotage training and recruitment efforts. Creating a massive global revolving door phenomenon is wasteful. Introducing nurses into dysfunctional health systems—ones that are not capable of retaining staff—is a nonsensical, frustrating exercise, likely to fail.

Yet, in country after country, conditions continue to produce shortages of nurses willing to work in nursing. The Norwegian Nurses Association believes there is no real shortage of nurses in their country. Surveys confirm that a considerable number of nurses working outside the profession or employed part-time would be prepared to fill vacant nursing positions if improvements in salaries and working conditions were introduced.[110] In Ireland an estimated fifteen thousand qualified nurses and midwives are opting not to work in their profession. More than half of these have maintained their registration and could possibly be attracted back into active practice. The other half, nurses no longer registered and not working, represent an additional pool of potential recruits.[111] There are, therefore, approximately 10,500 nurse candidates that could return to fill the 1,000 vacant posts, as well as the 4,000 posts now filled by internationally recruited nurses. What the figures clearly demonstrate is what observer after observer has noted. Although we may not have a shortage of nurses per se, there exists a shortage of nurses willing to work for the current pay and under the working conditions on offer. For example, in South Africa there are 32,000 nurse vacancies in the public sector, and 35,000 registered nurses are either inactive or unemployed.[112]

Under- and overemployment may distort or even make it impossible for researchers to correctly calculate the actual numbers of nurses working in any health care system. Head counts (the number of individuals presently on the nursing register) are the most common supply figures provided. A comparison with the number of position vacancies gives a quick but superficial overview of the supply/demand status of a given country or locality. These figures do not, however, adequately portray the numbers of nurses employed who are working part-time or who work significant hours overtime. In theory a group of a hundred nurses working half-time will fill the equivalent of fifty full-time positions. A group of a hundred nurses each working ten hours of overtime per week will be covering the requirements for 125 full-time positions. Head counts and vacancy figures need to be converted into full-time employment equivalents if they are to be helpful in determining the existing employment coverage and potential expansion of a given workforce.

When one considers statistics tallying the supply of nurses, the inefficient use of nurses may also create a false impression of where nurses actually work and what they actually do. Increasingly reliable data demonstrate that nurses are assigned tasks that do not require their advanced skills. The percentage of time spent by clinical nurses on management and support-worker responsibilities has greatly increased, a trend exacerbated by the downsizing exercises of recent years. In the United States, Canada, and Germany, Aiken and colleagues found,

> many nurses reported spending time performing functions that did not call upon their professional training, while care activities requiring their skills and expertise were often left undone. For example, the percentage of nurses who reported cleaning rooms or transporting food trays or patients ranged from roughly one-third to more than two-thirds. At the same time, a number of tasks that are markers of good nursing care, such as oral hygiene and skin care, teaching, and comforting patients, were frequently reported as having been left undone.

The reports from North America indicate also that front-line nursing management (nurse manager) positions have been cut and that top nursing management positions (the chief nursing officer level of management) have been eliminated in a number of hospitals. These findings imply that in addition to having responsibility for more patients, staff nurses might also have to take on more responsibilities for managing services and personnel at the unit level, which take time away from direct patient care.[113]

James Buchan makes the point that "shortage is not just about numbers but about how the health system functions to enable nurses to use their skills effectively."[114] Nursing workforce experts now make the distinction between a nursing crisis and a nurse shortage. Stephen Lewis, special UN envoy for AIDS in Africa, believes that "the extent of shortage will only be known when nurses spend all their time nursing. . . . nurses spend much of their time doing things that should be delegated to others and not enough of their time doing what they are educated to do. . . . Achieving a proper division of labor that respects and maximizes professionals' competencies will make the healthcare system more effective and efficient. It will also create a better motivated and contented workforce."[115] Hospital cutbacks in support personnel, such as patient transporters and food delivery workers, can lead to a major misuse of scarce nursing resources, often exaggerated during the weekends when nurses find themselves substituting for a wide range of other personnel.

Waiting Lists

In industrialized countries with national health services, the increasing length of waiting lists gives an indication of the growing demand for services that cannot be immediately provided. The time it takes to access health services has become a major political campaign issue in Canada and the United Kingdom. Promises to shorten the lists become a central message of party platforms. According to a recent OECD working paper, waiting times for elective (nonurgent) surgery are a main health policy concern in approximately half of its members (industrialized countries). Waiting times can lead to deterioration in health, loss of productivity or independence, and extra costs—all producing dissatisfaction for patients and the general public. Waiting lists become a type of rationing of health services, determining who will get needed treatment and when. They are a means of equilibrating supply and demand, but are quickly rejected by patients if waiting times are considered excessively long.

A common response has been to introduce strategies that shorten waiting lists: for example, employing more staff, creating comprehensive "one-stop" health centers, streamlining administrative procedures, and introducing computer technology. But since consumer demand responds positively to a reduction of waiting times, demand increases soon after the improvements are registered, and waiting times are once again at unacceptably high levels.[116] This becomes a perpetual, upwardly spiraling increase of demand and renewed initiatives to reduce waiting times. Recognizing the limited numbers of available national staff, growth has depended on opening the doors to internationally recruited nurses and outsourcing services to foreign private health care providers, such as Netcare (South Africa). The shortage of nurses is affecting national politics as well as the health industry, both private and public.

International Recruitment

International recruitment has become a strategy of choice when industrialized countries confront the challenges outlined above. Traditionally, recruitment of migrant workers, such as seasonal agricultural workers, has been seen as a quick solution to periodic labor shortages. For those involved, migration was mostly opportunistic or based on individual motivation and personal contacts.[117] However, the search for labor has now become a highly organized war for talent and skills, and it includes nurses.

Having exhausted many of the traditional sources of new recruits in the North, industrialized countries began to explore other potential suppliers, notably the countries in the South. Emerging diseases decimating populations in the South, however, have exacerbated the serious depletion of the nursing workforce brought on by public-sector restructuring. In Malawi and Zambia "five to sixfold increases in health worker illness and death rates have reduced personnel, and increased stress, overwork and fears for personal safety in remaining staff. . . . In southern Africa, the HIV/AIDS epidemic is likely to have been the most important determinant of non-migratory human resource attrition from the workforce."[118] According to the ILO, "the health service in South Africa reports that, between 1997 and 2001, 14 percent of staff (principally nursing staff) died as a result of AIDS. It is estimated that Botswana will have lost 17 percent of its health-care workers between 1999 and 2005, and if health care workers are not treated, the proportion of those dying as a result of HIV/AIDS may reach 40 percent by 2010."[119] A study from South Africa shows that the dramatic upsurge of patient volume due to HIV/AIDS and related opportunistic infections (e.g., tuberculosis) has increased worker burnout to the extent that the average number of days off work for nurses grew from forty-two in 1998 to fifty-eight in 2001.[120] Looking at the whole continent of Africa, HIV/AIDS is estimated to be the cause of between 19 and 53 percent of all deaths of health employees in the public sector. Some experts estimate that a person living with AIDS may be away from work for up to half the time of their final year of life.[121] Caring for ill family members or dependents and attending funerals are also known to contribute to worker absenteeism.

The documented transmission of HIV/AIDS at the workplace has been very low. The evidence indicates that the risk of transmission from infected patients to health care workers is greater than from infected workers to patients. Up to June 1999, only 102 documented cases of HIV transmission after occupational exposure from patients were reported worldwide.[122] It is difficult to make the distinction and quantify occupational HIV transmission in countries where the prevalence of HIV/AIDS is high in the general population. Nurses tend to have similar rates of infection, and this may be close to 40 percent in some sub-Saharan countries. For example, Swaziland's latest national survey of AIDS infection in adults found a rate of 38.6 percent, but a recent UNICEF survey found rates as high as 49.5 percent in some areas for women aged nineteen to thirty. Botswana's infection rate is 37.5 percent.[123] Several countries in Africa are in the same range (Uganda, 30 percent; Zambia, 40 percent) while others have very different profiles (Senegal, 1.43 percent; Nigeria, 5.8 percent; Kenya, 6.6 percent). In four South African provinces, 15.7 percent of health workers employed in the public and private health facilities were living with HIV/AIDS in 2002. This figure mirrors the HIV/AIDS prevalence seen in the general public, which that same year was 15.6 percent. Among younger health workers (aged eighteen to thirty-five) the risk was as high as 20 percent.[124]

While Africa has attracted the most attention, the rapid expansion of the HIV/AIDS epidemic in Eastern Europe and Central Asia is alarming. The number of people living with HIV has risen dramatically in just a few years—reaching an estimated 1.4 million at the end of 2004, more than a ninefold increase in less than ten years. While the overall numbers of infections are considered to be low, HIV transmission is occurring at a brisk rate and threatens an epidemic of dramatic proportions similar to that of southern Africa if not addressed immediately.[125]

After analyzing the statistics available from Africa, Barbara Stilwell, who works for the World Health Organization, found that the nurses' rate of attrition by death from HIV/AIDS in some countries may be as high as the emigration rate.[126] In countries like Zambia, where the prevalence rate is 40 percent, the health sector may be expected to lose 40 percent of its present nurses within the next ten years. The international attention that the tremendous loss of nurses from HIV/AIDS has attracted does not, however, seem to create the level of concern generated by international migration. The situation is very worrisome and begs at least the same amount of discussion and strategic action, if not more. The threat to personal safety that nurses and their families experience in the South certainly plays a significant role in nurse migration.

The pulling of nurses from other countries is both reinforced and, at times, initiated by a sophisticated international recruitment machinery that developed in the late 1990s. Attractive packages are assembled to take advantage of the range of migration push and pull factors that are likely to influence nurses' decision to migrate. Recruitment bonuses, scholarships, and free trips entice nurses to work abroad. The press has reported "golden hellos" in the United States of $35,000 for newly recruited nurses.[127] Seny Lipat, past president of the Philippine Nurses Association of America, explains that hospitals in Texas have offered bonuses of up to $50,000, granted over the course of the first complete year of employment. While this may be exceptional, many hospitals offer newly employed nurses between $1,000 and $7,500 as a recruitment bonus, sometimes followed by additional payments of $500 for every month on the job. One hospital offers a $2,100 retention bonus every six months. This means that nurses are actually paid for not taking another job. Other hospitals have decided to offer additional benefits such as access to a leased car, $7,500 toward a house down payment, a $10,000 scholarship, or an all-expenses-paid trip to Hawaii.[128]

Presenting a nurse to an interested employer or recruitment agency can lead to an attractive bonus, similar to a finder's fee. For example, in the Philippines a staff nurse or nurse educator who convinces a new graduate or colleague to sign an employment contract to work abroad may be rewarded with a $1,000 check. This represents ten months of salary for many nurses in the Philippines. With every five nurses recruited to the United States, one recruitment agency offers the "finder" a free return trip to the United States in addition to the accumulated $5,000 fees. One hospital in Nevada has begun giving current employees a finder's fee of a thousand dollars for referring nurses, an additional thousand dollars if the nurse stays six months, and a thousand dollars more if the recruit stays a year.[129] Clearly the competition for nurses has increased the stakes to a level never before seen.

Barriers to Migration

No matter how hard a nurse is either pushed or pulled toward migration, she or he will inevitably confront significant barriers to relocation in another country. The expense of re-qualification and physical transfer, the need to learn a new language and different clinical practices, and the costly and time-consuming immigration procedures are all challenges that must be surmounted. The difficulty embedded in the re-qualification process and language requirements cannot be underestimated.

The recognition of qualifications and competencies is often a long, frustrating, and expensive process. While the procedure may be streamlined in certain cases for immigration purposes, it is nevertheless a very important professional and public health measure.

Some trade policy experts claim that the re-qualification process of migrant nurses is primarily a measure that protects the nursing profession rather than the patients under the nurses' care. It limits the numbers of nurses, and this in turn means that, according to the laws of supply and demand, salaries will be kept to a maximum level. While this aspect certainly cannot be ignored, patient safety is—or should be—the ultimate goal of re-qualification when screening internationally recruited nurses. Nurses have four fundamental responsibilities: to promote health, to prevent illness, to restore health, and to alleviate suffering.[130] Careful screening of those who would use the title of nurse is critical to ensure that patients receive safe care and quality service, delivered by clinicians who have the appropriate levels of competence, knowledge, and skills.

Without doubt the verification of qualifications also protects the nurse who has personally and financially invested in acquiring professional status. The title of registered nurse permits access to professional nursing positions with their corresponding rewards and benefits. Trade and economic advisers, however, consider streamlining title verification and the reduction of qualification criteria in order to facilitate and ensure the international movement of labor. Their legal tools are geared almost exclusively toward trade and migration, not to patient safety, which creates a tension between health care professionals and strategic policy makers.

A second major hurdle to migration, communication, is also a cornerstone of patient care. In addition to the verification of qualifications, done by résumé submission, interview, exam, or supervised clinical placement, many countries impose a language test on foreign nurses who wish to practice in their country. Vital communication needs to take place between patients and care providers. Patients convey their concerns, describe their pain and symptoms, and report changes in their health status to professionals who, at a sheer minimum, must be able to understand what is being communicated. Nurses and patients need to work together to plan a viable course of treatment, and they must be able to converse if the nurse is to monitor the patient's progress. Nurses must be able to speak with one another and with other clinicians and health care workers. Moreover, they need language fluency to communicate under stress and duress, for example, when delivering emergency services or during resuscitation procedures. Even when people share the same mother tongue, they may have different accents and use different colloquialisms, slang, and conversational shortcuts, all of which make comprehension more difficult. Adding to this is the challenge of speaking in a second (or third) language and using technical medical terms.

In today's world, communication is further complicated by the fact that a great deal of information gathering and care planning is done via the telephone. This represents a significant pitfall for the foreign nurse. When a nurse cannot register someone's body language or verify something in writing, she loses an essential support to verbal communication. The absence of this kind of automatic and unconscious checking for comprehension may lead to misunderstandings that go uncorrected. Errors often occur when verbal orders are given over the phone, even when nationals are involved at both ends of the conversation. Clearly, this margin of error will increase if one of the parties is not completely fluent in the language used at the workplace.

In fact, many nurses have reported difficulty in managing telephone conversations in a foreign language, both with families and colleagues. In some cases, this has caused tension within the nursing team. Acknowledging their limitations, foreign nurses may systematically refuse to answer the telephone or ask others to take responsibility for work-related phone conversations. While this may seem a small favor to ask, nurses who are fluent in the language of their country are often so overburdened with high workloads of their own that they may not welcome the additional task.

Language is such a difficult hurdle that it often prevents nurse migration. Consider the example of the European Union. Since 1977 professional regulations called the Nursing Directives of the European Union have imposed on member states a set of minimum standards of nursing education for the practice of general nursing. First-level registered general nurses from the original fifteen EU nations have free mobility within the union, and these directives guarantee mutual recognition of nursing qualifications.[131] There has, however, been very little international migration between EU countries, although re-qualification and work permit requirements are waived. In fact, according to a recent report on UK international recruitment the overall contribution of EU nurses has decreased in percentage as well as absolute numbers over recent years.

Several reasons have been given for the low rate of nurse mobility within the European Union: limited oversupply, member state infringements (for example, lack of compliance recognizing qualifications issued in other countries), doubts that foreign qualifications really meet the criteria, and discriminatory practices. But there is consensus that one of the main barriers remains language.[132]

Language appears to influence the choice of destination country. English-speaking nurses from developing countries will tend to migrate to English-speaking industrialized countries—the United States, Canada, the United Kingdom, Australia. Francophone African nurses will more often migrate to industrialized regions where French is the mother tongue, like France, Belgium, and Québec. Portuguese-speaking nurses in Africa, from Angola or Mozambique, tend to migrate to Portugal. As the pool of nurses in the source countries shrinks, new countries are approached and traditional language channels are no longer considered absolute. The introduction of Cuban nurses in Botswana and Chinese nurses in Ireland is proof of the permeability and expansion of traditional language links.

The new world of nurse migration brings numerous challenges and opportunities to individuals and health care systems. To understand them one must move beyond the statistics to look at the experiences of some of the nurses who are moving around the globe today. What are the trade-offs they make? Are the social costs worth the economic gains? How are they greeted when they enter a new workplace, a new country? Where do they live, what do they see, and most important, how do they feel?

2. The Human Face of Nurse Migration

In June 2004 an elegant and charismatic fifty-seven-year-old woman, barely five feet tall, stood in front of hundreds of nurses in Minneapolis to receive one of the American Nurses Association's most prestigious awards, the Honorary Human Rights Award. Lolita B. Compas, a nurse who migrated to the United States more than thirty years earlier, was honored for her "outstanding commitment to human rights" and for exemplifying "the essence of nursing's philosophy about humanity."

Compas, who is the president of the New York State Nurses' Association (NYSNA), a state affiliate of the ANA, has over the years championed the rights of migrant nurses, fought their exploitation and abuse, and helped them navigate the difficult journey from their culture of origin to life in the United States. When Compas reaches out to migrant nurses, her assistance is based on the insight that can arise only from personal experience.

As Compas tells it, her story is an almost textbook case of Filipino migration. A Roman Catholic who was raised in what was then a small town fifty miles from Manila, Compas was the seventh of eleven children. Her mother stayed at home to take care of the family and her father worked in various jobs—as a jeep driver, a foreman on a construction site, and a book-keeper. Although neither of Compas's parents had been to college, their highest priority was to make sure their children received a college education. And indeed, all of the children graduated from university. Early on, Compas learned that life was about taking care of other people.

In fact, understanding her obligation to the family determined Compas's career. She had originally wanted to be a nun. But going into the convent would not have allowed Compas to fulfill her family responsibilities. Nursing, to which she had always felt drawn, was a way to serve others, get an education, forge a career, and help her family as well. Compas went to a top nursing school in the Philippines. "After graduation, my mother told me that it was now my turn to help the family by contributing money for the education of my younger brothers and sisters," she recalls. But that was only possible if Compas left the Philippines.

Faced with the same set of obligations, an older sister had gone to the United States and was working at Cabrini Hospital in Manhattan. Moving to New York therefore seemed to be a logical step. Compas's own skill and knowledge, along with the support network she quickly established at Cabrini Hospital, helped her move up the career ladder.

Over the years, as Compas moved from staff nurse to management to clinical education, she became known as a person to whom migrant nurses could turn for advice. Always energetic, she became a union activist when the NYSNA organized her hospital. She eventually became a member of the union negotiating committee, then its chairperson. While getting a master's degree in nursing, she also became active in the Philippine Nurses Association of America (PNAA).

"During the massive shortage of the eighties, the entire city of New York, particularly the Health and Hospital Corporation, was recruiting nurses by the hundreds from the Philippines. American recruiters were partnering with Filipino recruiters back home," she explains. "I would get calls from chairpersons at different facilities represented by NYSNA. These people would suddenly have forty to fifty Filipino nurses in their orientation programs. American nurses were unprepared to handle members of another culture in such large numbers." Working with another Filipino nurse, Priscilla Santayana, Compas developed an orientation program that introduced American nurses to Philippine culture and history. With her NYSNA and PNAA colleagues, she fought against the exploitation of migrant nurses.

Although Compas has returned often to the Philippines, she knows she will never go back permanently. Nonetheless, she is deeply concerned about conditions in her native country. "The situation for many people, including nurses," she says, "makes immigration not a choice but a necessity. The failure to improve those conditions leads to a depopulation of professionals that is causing havoc in the Philippine health system." Of her ten brothers and sisters, not a single one lives in the Philippines. It took eighteen years for all of them to come, but they are all in the United States.

Lolita Compas's story is one of successful nurse migration. Although few migrant nurses have received awards or been elected or appointed to leadership positions, many feel that despite difficult adjustments, their experiences have, on balance, been positive. For others, the road they traveled has been an endless obstacle course and their economic or professional goals have not been achieved. Whether the migrants' stories end positively or not, we should listen closely. They show us the human face of migration, often veiled by bewildering statistics, economic jargon, and legalistic policy prescriptions.

It is impossible to capture the life experiences that propel millions of nurses across the globe. By considering a few individual nurses who represent the categories outlined in the previous chapter, we can, however, gain some understanding of their challenges and motivations.

The Adventurer

A small but significant group of nurse migrants search for adventure or long for a change of scenery, mission, or pace. For example, Leah Daniels*, a Canadian nurse, combined a desire for change and adventure with a sense of mission. When her husband was offered a job that took the family to Africa, Daniels was happy to go along, for she was interested in exploring new political and cultural realities. Once in southern Africa, she worked with colleagues from many different disciplines. With their support and encouragement, she became involved in a variety of different projects.

The work she did in Africa bore no resemblance to her former responsibilities as a Canadian emergency room nurse. "I was now working at community level, engaging with players within civil society and government," Daniels told me. "It presented a valuable opportunity to learn about grass roots initiatives, the politics of health and health care, and the richness and potential of social action." The most formidable "surprise" Daniels remembered was an intense longing for her former position as an emergency care nurse. "After six months, I suddenly found myself missing the familiarity of the professional environment, my colleagues, the challenges of the clinical environment. I hadn't expected the feelings would be as acute as they were."

Within months, Daniels integrated this new world made up of nationals and expatriates. "I was generally treated very well, perhaps too well at times, which I thought was due to my nationality, skin color, and disposition," she recalled. In spite of her circle of friends and colleagues, Daniels struggled with loneliness and isolation. Her husband's work required far more travel than they had expected, and he would be gone for weeks at a time. "I wrote voraciously to my friends and family, describing the sounds and textures of Africa," she said. "For the first time in my life, I was living within an environment where my middle-class standard of living stood out as the exception to the standards of the majority of the population. The spirit of community in Africa is far richer than in my postindustrial country. It took some time to adjust to this new life and unfamiliar culture."

After twelve years Daniels returned to Canada, this time as a newly divorced single parent. Reentry, she says, was difficult. "The challenges I faced were entirely unexpected. I returned older, to a different work environment and a hugely changed social network." Daniels found that the treasure trove of experiences she brought back from Africa were of little interest to Canadians. "I felt intensely alone. One's community is of primary importance. I think I took it for granted, until I returned to Canada to find it had dissolved."

The call of adventure does not always involve exotic or faraway lands. Rachel Turner* was also eager to travel. Turner, a university graduate now in her thirties, moved to the United States after working as a nurse for two years in a Toronto hospital. Although many Canadian nurses go south to earn more money, the chance to have "the adventure of my life" was her primary motivation; the US nursing shortage was the pull that made the journey possible. Since 1994 the US government has allowed Canadian nurses to go to the United States with relative ease, and they enjoyed benefits unavailable to most other migrant nurses. "Approximately 15,000 Canadians work in the United States under the North America Free Trade Agreement on what is known as a TN (Trade NAFTA) visa, which is renewed annually," Turner explained.

Having her work permit, Turner fulfilled the professional accreditation requirements and was given a license to practice nursing. She has found her work in a large teaching hospital in Philadelphia to be the adventure she was seeking. "Most of my shocking experiences with the American health care system have been due to my attempts to find a health care provider for myself. In Canada, because we have universal health care, anybody can go to see a doctor. There are no qualifiers and you don't have to pay out-of-pocket cash." She found it disturbing that so many working families and children in the United States have no easy access to health promotion and treatment services. And Turner was amazed that her American colleagues had so many misconceptions about the Canadian health care system. "Americans believe that in Canada people have to wait a long time to get tests and services," she explains, "but in Canada, just like in the US, waits depend on volume." As Turner's experience suggests, exposure to different health systems and their methods of work can transform an adventure into a useful learning experience, dispelling myths along the way.

Changing attitudes toward migrants after the attacks of September 11 are making it more difficult for migrant nurses to work in the United States. Indeed, recent changes in US government policy illustrate that nurses, like other migrant workers, are vulnerable to international events and political shifts. Prior to 9/11, working in the United States was so easy that many Canadian nurses who live in border states like Maine or Michigan had, for years, lived in Canada while traveling to work in the United States. The situation is now very different. Competing interests in cross-border trade, patient safety, professional regulation, and immigration/security concerns have heightened tensions and resulted in new policies that affect migrant nurses. The US government recently announced that the days of the special relationship between Canadian nurses and the US health care system have ended. Like all other foreign-educated nurses, Canadians are now required to take the US licensing exam. Turner explains:

> Even though we've already passed a Canadian board exam, possess a US license, and have been practicing under that license, and even though the country is in the middle of a nursing shortage that we were hired to relieve, they are asking us to write the board exam. It's very stressful. Many of us are not new graduates. The licensing exam is easier for people who have just gotten out of school. But think about someone who's been out of school for ten years, or even twenty years. She's a specialist in orthopedics, and she has to go back and write a general exam that covers all the nursing domains. She will have to devote a great deal of time studying for the exam while continuing to work, and she will have to spend a lot of money.

The United States is also encouraging Canadian nurses to apply for green cards—that is, permanent resident status. But many Canadian nurses do not want to become permanent residents; they just want to work in the United States temporarily and then go home. "To get a green card, you need to get a lawyer," Turner adds. "That alone costs about $5,000." Canadians who were on a TN visa had to rethink their motivations for working in the United States. They needed to decide whether or not it was worth staying. "This," she predicts, "may have a big impact on how many nurses decide to go to the United States in the future."

Many Canadian nurses emigrated to the United States because of the dearth of full-time jobs back home. The present Canadian nursing shortage, however, has gained the attention of the public and, finally, the politicians. Salaries have gone up and there are more permanent full-time jobs. US salaries may no longer be so much better, and Canadian nurses may enjoy better health care benefits at home. Turner fears that the kind of international experiences that helped her grow professionally may suffer. The nurse seeking adventure may not be prepared to become an economic migrant.

The Economic Migrant

Although there are no firm figures that tell us how many of the globe's estimated twelve million nurses migrate for economic reasons, financial considerations probably predominate and definitely influence the decision for a vast majority. Nurses worldwide generally share one common reality: they are relatively underpaid and awarded poor benefits. As mentioned, equal pay for work of equal value is not a reality for nursing. In Geneva the salary of the community nurse was sixty-four Swiss francs per hour in 1995, whereas a skilled technician—for example, a washing machine repairman—was paid one hundred francs per hour. The wage comparison with teachers, social workers, and policeman is almost always unfavorable for nurses. In several countries including Switzerland, Canada, the United States, and Sweden nurses are resorting to equal-opportunity legislation to demand higher and comparable wages. The courts in many cases have seen the value of their arguments and have awarded significant wage hikes. In March 2005, UNISON settled the biggest ever equal pay award with North Cumbria Acute NSH Trust. According to the union, women working full-time earn, on average, 82 percent of the hourly earnings of men working full-time. These averages hide wider disparities, with part-time workers' pay stuck at just 60 percent of the hourly pay of men working full-time.[1] As many nurses work part-time, they face double discrimination. Equal-value claims were lodged for fifteen hundred women employed in fourteen different working categories, including nurses. Pay rates, hours of work, pension, weekend working rates, and sick pay were all included in the comparison, which showed that women were treated unfairly by the old pay system. Some of the women will receive up to fourteen years' back pay with interest, with each woman standing to gain between £35,000 and £200,000.

Where nurses have negotiated comparable salaries for new graduates, they are confronted with a phenomenon called "wage compression." The financial progression over the span of a career is not the same for all professions, and the nurse who is close to retirement age will earn far less than professionals in similar disciplines and length of service, even when starting salaries are identical. This is yet another battle in the search for equitable pay and working conditions.

In less-developed and in-transition countries a nurse may earn a salary that is under the poverty line. Imagine a hard-working professional, who has the knowledge, skills, and responsibility to make life-and-death decisions, working two jobs in order to have sufficient revenue to cross the poverty line. Salaries are low. Permanent positions may be unavailable—frozen by recent health-sector reforms. The poorer the country the nurse comes from, the more likely it is that family needs—not personal or professional ones—will strongly influence career choices. Men have always considered how they will support themselves, a spouse, and children as they weigh career options. Women of today increasingly make a similar calculation.

When Maricar Baez* thought about her future, she knew it included helping her family. However, although she was working full-time, her salary was not enough to pay her rent. Her father was obliged to supplement her monthly income. This, she felt, was not acceptable. She began to consider migration to the United States as a solution. Looking around, Baez realized that she was one of the only nurses of her graduating class still in the Philippines.

Baez passed the pre-licensing test given by the US-based Commission on Graduates of Foreign Nursing Schools and applied directly to the Hospital Corporation of America (HCA). The hospital company sent a recruiter to interview Baez in the Philippines and hired her on the spot. The HCA owned hundreds of smaller hospitals around the United States and offered her a list of possible employment sites. She chose New Mexico.

Baez passed her US licensing exam within the first six months of her arrival in the country. Although the HCA made the recruitment and moving process as easy as possible, adjusting to the new environment was difficult. "I had been working at the intensive care unit in the Philippines, but in New Mexico I was put on the night shift in the labor and delivery ward on an understaffed unit," Baez explains. "I was very young and the only registered nurse on the unit. They required you to be perfect and to do everything— mopping and sterilization as well as delivering babies." While the work was hard, discrimination made it unbearable.

> I felt the racism. The patient cases were often difficult. There was one crazy night that I will always remember. I had already had fifteen or sixteen deliveries and I was exhausted. A woman came in and I delivered her twin premature babies. My shift had finished long ago—I was often working overtime and never getting paid for it. All I wanted to do was go to bed. The day shift nurse started yelling at me using abusive racist language. She said that I could not leave until I had cleaned the instruments. I had had enough. I talked back and went home. I was called in by the director and asked to apologize. I refused and explained what had happened. I was not made to apologize, but the whole experience had been a nightmare.

Baez stayed until the end of her contract, but she did not renew it. Encouraged by friends as well as aunts and cousins in New York City, she decided to join them. Baez found New York somewhat familiar—"almost like Manila." Nonetheless, she had to cope with one principal difficulty—"as a migrant nurse, I felt the lack of support. I got sick," she remembers. "Everybody works. Everybody's busy. I have lots of friends but it's not the same. There is no substitution for family."

On balance, she feels the experience has been a positive one. "The salary is good—it covers all my expenses. You earn money and learn to be independent. Family clans can be very big and often decide for you. This way you can live freely. I go home every year, and with my savings my family started a business ten years ago. They live comfortably. I continue to send money home. It is my turn to give something back." Not only to her family and country of origin. She proudly states that as a migrant nurse, "you help America care for their sick."

As Baez moves into her mid-forties, she also understands that she will "not be able to nurse forever." Her plans are "to retire early and go home." Something she may be able to do because her economic gamble has paid off.

Namjoo Chung* also had a positive experience as an economic immigrant from Korea. In the beginning, for Chung nursing was all about economics. Although she had always wanted to be a physician, medical school was unaffordable for a family with five sisters and brothers. Nursing became an attractive alternative. After World War II the Scandinavian development fund established and financed a South Korean nursing school, whose courses were taught in English. The school quickly gained an excellent reputation and was considered a model for the nation. Chung applied and received a merit scholarship. Even though choosing nursing meant giving up the dream that she would become a physician, she quickly became the envy of her community because the school was known to facilitate employment in the United States.

In her final year of studies, a recruiter came to her school and interviewed Chung. Employment in the United States promised her the opportunity to be independent, financially self-sufficient, and career oriented. Chung was promised a good salary, help in adjusting to the move, and fully paid postgraduate education. She chose to work in Detroit.

Chung's travel expenses were paid; she lived in a clean nurses' dormitory that had a night security guard. Her colleagues helped orient her to the neighborhood, and the director of nursing was generous to foreign nurses, often inviting them to social events. The hospital staff filed all the immigration papers.

In order to obtain the permanent work permit (green card), Chung was asked to take the licensing exam shortly after arrival. She was the only one from her group of newly recruited nurses to pass on the first try. Although her nursing studies had been in English, there was, nonetheless, a serious language barrier on the ward. To help her overcome this hurdle, her employer hired a private tutor, and she was given lessons for seven months. Her first-year evaluation was excellent, and she was transferred to the intensive care unit. With opportunities for free continuing education and internal transfers, Chung managed to upgrade her skills in critical care cardiology and pediatrics. She went on to get her master's in clinical practice.

Even with help from her employer, Chung says, "I struggled those first years. There were some surprises. For example, I had never seen a black person and I found them frightening. The patients were so much bigger than I was. At the time, I weighed ninety pounds." Another thing she had to confront was jealousy from some of her American coworkers. "I was not aware of any discrimination at first. There was, however, much jealousy, although most of the support I received," she admits, "was from US nurses."

Perhaps some of the ill will stemmed from her willingness to work longer hours than her colleagues, both to prove herself and earn extra money for her family. "I worked harder and longer hours, sometimes with no overtime pay. But the supervisor heard of my work, and I got rewarded with paid further education. I volunteered to go where US nurses didn't want to go. I worked double shifts. I would rather work just to keep busy as I had no social life. I learned a lot about myself." She paused. "I realized that I wanted to get married before I died. I returned to South Korea, got engaged and then married a man I had known before I left for the States." Her husband was then going to medical school, and the two went back to the United States after his graduation so he could do his internship. When he finished, it was time to make another decision. Should they stay or return to South Korea? "If it were not for my husband, I would have stayed in the US," Chung explains.

Readjusting to life in South Korea was not easy. "It is difficult to readjust. Korean and US thinking are like oil and water. My husband prefers life in Korea because a man is more comfortable. When we were in the US, my husband helped me with the household chores. Since our return, this no longer happens." Chung's case highlights the gender dilemmas and paradoxes that so often underlie nurse migration. When on their own, nurse migrants from less-developed countries often find a degree of independence they would never have at home. The status of the female migrant nurse and her marital relationship may change, however, if she and her husband decide to return home.

Chung soon became involved in lifelong learning programs with the local university and worked with several organizations to facilitate the migration of South Korean nurses. She is a pioneer in Asia, where she has helped to establish innovative international partnerships. Chung recommends the migration experience. Although it was not easy, the multitude of learning opportunities as well as the exposure to different cultures, values, and thinking made it all worthwhile, she says. The only incentive that would have kept her in South Korea in her youth was more money.

Although Chung and Baez ultimately feel their economic gamble paid off, not all economic migrants have positive experiences. Gladys Reyes*, a Panamanian, wanted to be a nurse ever since she was a child. She loves her profession but is very disillusioned because of the many injustices she has witnessed over the years. As a single parent with two young children, Reyes found herself in very difficult financial circumstances and unable to provide for her family as she would like. After consulting with her children and close family members, Reyes made the decision to migrate from Panama to Italy. She hoped to improve her financial situation and become familiar with another culture. Information on employment opportunities was readily available through colleagues and family members who already had experience working in Italy. Reyes was offered an attractive recruitment package—accommodation, travel expenses, and a better salary. With the support of her family, she decided to move.

Although Reyes had fifteen years of employment in the same health facility in Panama, the administration refused to give her leave without pay. When she resigned from her job, she forfeited all her acquired benefits and gave up any guarantee that she would have a job waiting for her when she returned. Reyes felt she had no choice, and finally left Panama.

Once in Italy, in spite of better living and working conditions, Reyes quickly realized she was earning less than Italian nurses and yet assigned the same tasks. When she complained about this, nothing was done to correct the injustice. She also discovered undercurrents of resentment. Italian nurses sometimes considered foreign nurses with better academic preparation a threat to their career advancement.

Perhaps the biggest trauma Reyes faced was leaving her children behind. Indeed, what most distressed her was that this personal sacrifice of hers almost seemed futile. She sent money home, but her family mismanaged it, debts were not repaid, and they lost everything. This led to serious family conflicts that remain hard to resolve. Reyes says she now wishes her children had migrated with her and cautions her colleagues to be wary of entrusting money to anyone else, even to family members.

Reyes is now a return migrant back in Panama. The situation for nurses in her country is not promising. She has not yet been able to find employment and once again is looking for opportunities to migrate. Reyes looks back on her migration to Italy as a positive experience. "I have matured. I have learned to value life," she adds. Reyes feels she cannot afford to retire in Panama, and despite her difficulties in Italy she plans to go back there in search of a better life, but this time with her children.

The economic migrants discussed above came from developing countries and went to industrialized countries. But nurses also move between industrialized nations—going from one to another in search of better pay, professional development, and better working conditions. Restructuring initiated in the 1980s and 1990s in Canada, the United Kingdom, and the United States resulted in downsized health facilities, reduced permanent nurse employment opportunities, and at times lowered wages.

Elizabeth Hom*, a thirty-two-year-old Chinese-Canadian nurse, is one of the migrants driven away from her native Montreal by poor working conditions, the desire for an adventure, and the lure of better pay in another country. After graduating from nursing school in 1992, Hom says she was unable to find permanent full-time work. After five years of being on call for varying shifts, she finally got a full-time job on a surgical unit but found the working conditions very stressful. According to Hom, the chronic understaffing in Québec hospitals meant she was taking care not only of more patients but of patients with more intense needs.

From a friend who had gone to Switzerland a couple of years earlier, Hom learned that their health care system needed nurses and that Swiss employers offered better conditions and pay than in Canada. In the monthly French magazine *Infirmière*, which is available to all nurses in Québec, she found an ad from a recruiting agency that works specifically with a hospital in Lausanne. When she called the recruiter at their Québec office, she discovered that she could even be interviewed in Montreal. Hom learned that the Swiss would recognize her license, but as an Anglophone she would be required to prove proficiency in French.

Hom was very happy with the conditions she found in Switzerland. "We had time to sit down and speak with patients, which we rarely did in Québec. The hospital was in excellent condition. It was spotless." Hom was delighted with what she described as the Swiss health care system's commitment to patient service.

As an adventure, Hom says Switzerland proved to be a paradise for someone who enjoys the outdoors. But one of the most tantalizing bonuses was the money. "We were earning more than double what we earned in Québec. We had what is called the thirteenth salary, which means that in December we would get a whole extra month's salary, essentially getting paid twice, plus a Christmas bonus of five thousand Swiss francs, which is about five thousand Canadian dollars."

From Hom's point of view there was no downside. "I experienced no discrimination from Swiss nurses," she says, "maybe because there were so few of them. Almost all the nurses I worked with were from Québec or France. Even the assistant head nurse was from France. In fact, only 15 percent of the nurses I worked with were Swiss."

Blocked Opportunities for Career Advancement

For many nurses the motivating impulse for a move was simple—they could not meet their financial needs or support their families. Some could not get a job. If employed, the conditions were difficult and sometimes harsh. Some of these nurses had tried all their options, and it seemed there was nowhere else to go but away from home—often very far away. For other nurses, the issue was less stark but no less pressing. They had come to the end of a different road—that of professional advancement—and felt the only way they could move ahead in their career was to leave their country.

That was the conclusion Girija Ram* reached after he had worked for years in his home country of Mauritius. At the outset Ram was ambivalent about nursing. After graduating from high school he was looking for employment and found nursing. Eighteen months after starting his training, he left and joined the police force. "Six months later, I returned to nursing," he explains. "My experience (in the police) enabled me to appreciate this profession, which is a caring one. I stayed in nursing for my personal development, as it is a dynamic profession. It gave a sense to my life. I feel I am doing something marvelous by caring for sick people."

Ram advanced quickly in his profession. He applied for and received an international scholarship that financed his first post-basic degree in South Africa. After completing his nursing education and community nursing service studies, he eagerly returned to Mauritius to apply his newly acquired knowledge and skills. But he was not able to get a position teaching at the school of nursing.

"It was not only a question of salary and conditions of service which made me decide to migrate, although I must admit they were key elements. Other factors were equally important," Ram says. "I was unable to use my skills to teach nursing students and that was very frustrating. I definitely would have stayed if I had been successful in securing a job at the school of nursing."

The combination of blocked career advancement and economics was too powerful to overcome. Given the obstacles at home, the ease with which he realized his move was startling. Colleagues who had worked abroad fed him with a myriad of possible jobs in as many different countries. The Internet added to the seductive picture of better salaries and other fringe benefits. Migration offered him better working conditions such as weekend bonuses, night duty allowances, public holidays, and opportunities to develop his skills and move on academically.

Ram discussed his desire to move with his wife, who enthusiastically supported his decision. "My financial situation has greatly improved and my working conditions are better than in Mauritius. I have bought my own house and car. I am now studying for a bachelor of science in nursing practice with specialty in wound care at a UK university, and," he adds, "most of the program expenses are covered by my hospital." His wife, not a nurse, is also working. Both he and his wife believe that their children will have a better life in England. "In the future my daughter can have access to university in the UK. If I were still in Mauritius, I could never afford such opportunities for my family."

Because he hoped for a better quality of life and career advancement, Ram willingly shouldered the burdens of migration. "It is quite difficult to obtain a work permit, especially if you come from a third world country. The UK employer must prove that he has not been able to recruit nurses from the European countries. Because of government bilateral cooperation, second priority is attributed to the Philippines, then India, and finally other countries."

Financial obstacles were also significant. "You need to have enough money to survive in the UK for at least one month," he explains. "This is around £1,500 to £2,000. It is a huge sum for us Mauritian nurses—approximately seven months salary." Learning to adapt to another culture was also stressful. "In the UK, you have to stick to the three P's—protocols, procedures, and policies," he describes the process. "For many things, even if you know, you cannot venture. You have to wait for the doctor, and this can take a long time if it is not an emergency. It is not like in Mauritius where the nurse will carry out many of these duties."

Although Ram says he did not encounter overt discrimination in terms of promotion or career prospects, he found it difficult to be accepted at first. "You have to prove what you are worth. It takes time to integrate into the team and to adapt and learn the slang that may not be familiar to you. At the beginning, it was not easy being a foreigner and an Asiatic on top of that. People tend to have a certain prejudice against you. You have to persevere, and if you can prove that you are capable, they will accept you and your nightmare is over."

Ram insists that neither he nor most other migrant nurses would leave home if they had decent jobs, good pay, and opportunities for advancement. "Home is always best," he says bluntly. "You do feel this separation from your family, friends, working environment. It is a culture shock. No one would leave his native land if they were getting fair treatment."

What Ram most regrets is that what might have been only a temporary move has almost certainly turned into a permanent one. But the Ministry of Health's refusal to give him leave without pay makes it almost inevitable that he will be a permanent migrant. If he decided to return to Mauritius, he would most certainly lose all his seniority and would have to go back to the bottom of the professional ladder.

In resource-limited health systems, access to technological advances, skill development, and independent practice may remain a dream if the opportunity to practice abroad is refused or restricted. Exposure to nursing specialties, innovative methods of work, sophisticated equipment, and cutting-edge interventions, perhaps unavailable in their home countries, provides migrant nurses with an overview of new health care approaches as well as career advancement possibilities. Experience abroad often adds prestige to a nurse's curriculum vitae. For example, Troy Galang*, a community-based nurse in the Philippines, realized that his career was stagnating and that he would never be able to work autonomously. "All the books are written by Americans. Promotions at home automatically went to nurses who had work experience or degrees from the US. I started to investigate possibilities in the US. When the recruiter promised to pay all my expenses, I packed my bags and left. I never regretted my decision."

Quality of Life or Survival

For all these nurses the factors that pushed them out of their home countries were economic, professional, or personal. They left to seek jobs, promotions, opportunities for advancement, or adventure. For some of the world's migrant nurses, life in their home country is already filled with too much uncertainty and an endless series of challenges. Managing the daily realities within the workplace or outside may be fraught with risk—to their health and, at times, to their very life or the lives of loved ones.

Personal safety is a growing motivation for nurse migration. Nurses are subject to biological, chemical, physical, social, and sensory hazards. Slovakia has reported health care workers to be the third-largest group affected by occupational hazards. Malawi and Zambia report five- to sixfold increases in illnesses and deaths among health workers in recent years.[2] Swedish studies report similar findings. Cases of nurse burnout due to workplace-generated stress have significantly increased and generate serious concern. In the United States, nursing has the third-highest injury and illness rate, even before mining and construction.[3] In the light of the occupational hazards present in nurses' working environments, nursing has been categorized as one of the most dangerous professions.

In many countries, occupational health legislation is either nonexistent or unenforced. Where legislation exists, public health services are sometimes specifically excluded. This leaves employees particularly vulnerable to professional hazards.[4] With the HIV/AIDS epidemic, the need for protective measures and equipment to avoid transmission of disease at the health workplace has received greater attention. Nurses in financially constrained health systems are often confronted with the dilemma of caring for HIV/AIDS patients without basic equipment like gloves. In most of Africa "protection for health workers is considered to be rudimentary, and many cases are not covered by health or life insurance policies."[5] In one study the total absence of adequate protective measures and equipment when caring for HIV/AIDS patients was reported by 48 percent of interviewed health professionals in Senegal and Uganda.[6]

The number of reported cases of violence in the health sector is also increasing. In Sweden reported cases of workplace violence are much higher in the health sector (24 percent) than in other sectors such as retail trade, the police, education, transport, or banking (4–7 percent).[7] Once thought to be primarily a problem in industrialized countries, pioneering research undertaken by the Joint ILO/ICN/WHO/PSI Programme on Workplace Violence in the Health Sector documents that this is a worldwide challenge of epidemic proportions.[8] The two categories of violence—physical and psychological—exist in all countries to varying but unacceptably high degrees.

Stories of nurses who get nowhere when they raise the issue of workplace violence with management fuel the migratory stream. For example, one nurse in England was attacked during her shift in the emergency room. When she went to management to see if measures could be taken to ensure the personnel's safety, her managers told her that additional security was too expensive and therefore not cost-effective. Not surprisingly, she quit her job to find work where her personal safety was considered important.[9] The nurses she left behind got the message: the only safety option in this institution is to quit. No wonder nurses increasingly say that violence is a reason for leaving a given workplace, abandoning the profession, or migrating to another country where foreign coworkers are treated with more respect within a safer environment.

Violence occurring in nurses' external environment may also have a significant impact on decisions to migrate. Amnesty International has repeatedly denounced cases of health personnel being victimized in countries experiencing armed conflict or under oppressive regimes.[10] There is a clear link between civil unrest and migration. War is a major push factor in the migration of health professionals. Nurses and their families are not spared the trauma of forced and sudden migration.

For South African nurses, who must cope with the legacy of apartheid, personal safety is a major factor in their decision to migrate. Nurses like Mady van de Merve* struggle daily with quality-of-life issues that have become so pressing that they feel their very future or that of their children is endangered. Van de Merve entered nursing with high hopes. She thought it would be a satisfying career with many opportunities for specialty training and travel. Getting paid while studying made the profession additionally attractive. After getting an advanced diploma in community nursing, a master's in nursing education, and then a doctorate in nursing leadership, she found the major unresolved problems in health and nursing in South Africa demoralizing. The nursing shortages were escalating, turnover of staff no longer ensured continuity of care, morale was low, and workloads were high. In addition, safety was a growing concern.

"Personal safety for my family was a major incentive to move. I did not have the energy to deal with all those problems anymore and wanted to find something new and exciting to do," Van de Merve explained. After discussing things with her children, Van de Merve decided to migrate to Australia.

Australia was pulling South African nurses to its shores in often heavily attended recruitment seminars. "I attended some of the seminars offered by the migration agents," Van de Merve recalls. "I had enough points within the category of independent individual on the Australian migration points system and therefore did not need the sponsorship of a company. I had to pass the health exams and police clearance. A residency visa was then issued. When I received my visa, the kids and I spent six weeks in Australia before we finally came to a decision. Nothing would have made me stay in South Africa—we were totally convinced and still believe it was a good move. Although not easy! My brother still thinks I was totally crazy to migrate."

Some of her brother's skepticism was not unfounded. "When I moved, I found that many of the problems in health and nursing prevalent in South Africa also exist in Australia. I opted out and looked for a change in direction. I spent ten weeks looking for employment. Answering an ad for a teaching position, I was hired by a university to create a business leadership development course and program."

Although van de Merve found a job, she had to adjust to Australian culture. "Some colleagues were suspicious of the newcomer—especially because the newcomer was a foreigner. In Australia the principle of cutting down the tall poppy is very alive and can make life difficult," she elaborates. "This means that people will 'cut down to size' any person who is too successful." Learning to teach in a new culture was also difficult. Van de Merve had no experience with health care in Australia and thus could not use Australian examples in her teaching. She could not use her familiar textbooks, as the students proved not to be interested in South African examples. Even mastering classroom technology required an adjustment.

Van de Merve was initially so relieved to have left South Africa, she did not realize immediately how far she was from home. "I could not have foreseen the emotional impact or how hard it would really be, alone in a new country. I was the only adult in the family and had to make all the decisions and also build a life for us—basic practical things such as finding a doctor, dentist, the dry cleaners, a house, a school, et cetera. It was very scary."

Although Van de Merve has succeeded in creating a better life for herself and her children, she is well aware of the fact that what is good for her and her family is not good for South Africa and its health system. This she finds sad. "South Africa lost my knowledge and skills. I earned a good salary and therefore paid high taxes that they no longer get. I also would have contributed to the economy through day-to-day purchases. And they have lost the contribution that my kids could have made to the knowledge base and the economy." For Van de Merve, enduring what appeared to be intractable political and social problems, just so that South Africa might one day benefit, was not a valid choice.

Over the years, thousands of nurses have left their countries because their lives were in imminent danger of the political turmoil in their countries. In 1973, for example, Rosa Vasquez*, was caught in the aftermath of a coup d'état in Chile. The democratically elected socialist president, Salvador Allende, was assassinated and thousands of his supporters were jailed, killed, or disappeared. Identified as having prior links with the Allende regime, Vasquez received a series of death threats, which, given the political situation, were eminently credible. She learned that the embassy of Panama was recruiting nurses to relieve the critical nursing shortage in that country. The Panamanian government offered nurses a renewable one-year visa and paid for food and accommodation for the first year plus free air travel to the country. Vasquez consulted her father and he agreed that she should accept the offer and save her life. Once again safe and earning money, she arranged for her family to join her in Panama.

For Vasquez, migration was thus a particularly mixed blessing. "Migration had different contradictory effects on me and my family. On the one hand, we were given the possibility of life. I was able to save myself and later my family. On the other hand, I had to leave home and community, completely disrupt the normal cycle of my life—study, work, and starting a family in my native land. This demands a great deal of energy, sacrifice, and perseverance. I discovered strengths I didn't know I had."

Although glad to be alive and employed, she quickly discovered the downside of the one-year contracts. First, there was no relief from the job insecurities, and her years of service were excluded when calculating pension benefits. This discriminatory practice threatened her post-retirement financial viability. If she objected to the terms offered and refused to renew her contract, Vasquez not only faced being jobless, she faced being stateless.

Employers have often exploited this kind of situation to extract unfair terms from their employees. Isolated, far from home, and very vulnerable, migrant nurses have been bullied into accepting unfair contracts that bear no resemblance to the ones signed in their home countries.

Facing employment insecurities and personal vulnerability, Vasquez was fortunate to find help in the National Nurses Association of Panama. "They created a working group to negotiate for us. We received the needed support and these colleagues fought for the recognition of our years of service from the first year of employment in Panama. This lobbying had a direct impact on our salaries and pension benefits."

When Vasquez first went to Panama, she lived with the knowledge that she might never be able to go back to the country she loved. Asked if she would change anything, Vasquez thought for a moment and then answered that, of course, she would have preferred to leave Chile under different circumstances. A dramatic, life-threatening situation was the basis for her decision to migrate. Luckily, in her case, a life-preserving measure led to a happy ending. Although her experience was positive, she thought that the threat of death should not be a prime motivation for nurse migration. Nor should employers take advantage of nurse migrants, whatever their motive for migration. "If I could change anything, I wish that employers would establish fair relationships—clear and humane—with foreign personnel."

The Physician-Nurse

One of the most interesting new additions to the migrant nurse story is the physician who becomes a nurse. When it comes to the migration of skilled professionals, physicians have always been high on the list of those who emigrate. Widely cited although a bit dated, the famous Mejia study in 1976 estimated that 6 percent of physicians worldwide are migrants (compared to the 4 percent of nurses).[11] In some instances, physicians who migrate are able to get jobs in their fields either because they have had their qualifications automatically recognized in accordance with government mutual recognition agreements or because they have gone through the sometimes lengthy and costly national accreditation process of their destination country. In other instances, however, physicians find that getting licensed in another country is very arduous. As in nursing, the education received by the migrant physician is carefully evaluated as part of the re-qualification or credentialing process. In cases where the education is considered inferior, the license is refused. This process is most often independent from the immigration procedures that result in the granting of work permits. A foreign-educated physician who has a work permit but no license to practice medicine will likely end up employed in a job that does not utilize her or his medical education and skills. The physician driving a taxi or working as an auxiliary in a residential care facility may suddenly discover that becoming a nurse is an attractive and financially advantageous option. Nursing schools and health care administrators are discovering that physicians who want to retrain as nurses provide a stream of new students and recruits. The business interests of such ventures will be discussed in the next chapter.

Jean Fenelon, a Haitian physician granted political asylum in the United States after a failed political campaign in 1994, was picking oranges and selling water pumps to support a wife and three children. He learned about a physicians-to-nursing program offered by Florida International University and decided to enroll. Graduation from the program allowed Fenelon to return to health care in a challenging job in a cardiac unit. His journey is typical of a small but growing number of physicians. When he was forced into blue-collar work, the loss of self-esteem was almost unbearable. He acknowledged that for him and other physicians in nursing, "It's a second opportunity for us." But Fenelon admits that he and his fellow physicians had to struggle with their own prejudices against entering nursing, which was simultaneously seen as a demotion and a promotion. "Sometimes you have that feeling that once you are a doctor, you are always a doctor, but you need to see nursing as a promotion."[12] Like him, other graduates admitted that the program required a major change in thinking as well as acting. They felt a kind of professional "culture shock."

Education

Educational programs available abroad may be the only way to quench the thirst for further knowledge and broader horizons. Haile Kahsay* is enthusiastic when he recalls his first experience abroad and claims that it opened the doors to a whole new world. Kahsay, as a young nurse in Eritrea, accepted his first employment in a rural community—working relentlessly, having no days off as there was no one to relieve him. His idealism and determination were strengthened by a sincere desire to help save the world. Rewarded for his hard work, a scholarship took him to the United States and this golden opportunity changed his life. Kahsay couldn't wait to go back home. With his newly acquired knowledge and skills, he was now equipped to transmit his passion and teach his chosen profession, nursing, to others in his country. The experience abroad created a completely new and satisfying life for him and his family.

Personal goals may also include the enriching experience of teaching and supporting others in their pursuit of professional development. Having accumulated a certain level of expertise within a local or national context, moving abroad may be the natural progression which facilitates and extends the sharing of knowledge with others. Sora Park* welcomes the opportunity at the end of her nursing career to teach transcultural nursing in a neighboring country in Asia. Teaching in English, a foreign language in her destination as well as home countries, Park draws on her knowledge of international nursing policies and her years of experience with nursing practice in various countries around the world. Park promotes diversity in the nursing workforce as well as approaches to health care. Explaining the functions of international health and nursing organizations, she has the chance to broaden the horizons of her students, exposing them to new ideas, practices and policies.

Social Costs of Migration

As one listens to migrant nurses tell their stories, several important issues emerge. One is the social cost of migration. Some migrants pay a high price for a happy ending. Uprooting oneself, leaving one's family, community, and country of origin, and establishing oneself in a new country are all taxing events. The nurse who travels on her own and has no family or friends in her new land will, of course, suffer most. But even if a nurse has a support network, she has to establish new roots, learn different routines, interpret unfamiliar cultural signs and symbols, and draw a new life map. She has to deal with homesickness and with the added responsibility of providing not only for herself and her immediate family—if they are with her—but for any family left behind at home.

The importance of family and community is emphasized in practically all the stories. The social cost of separation from the family is paramount. Leaving the children behind is considered the most traumatic, closely followed by separation from the mother. As one nurse said, "Leaving my children was the most terrible thing I have ever had to do." Departing nurses count on mothers, husbands, or sisters to take care of their children. But there are no guarantees that these arrangements will work. Even if surrogate parents function well, asking women to place the economic survival of the family ahead of the bond with their children is a significant social demand.

Children pose a special challenge. In one scenario, the children are left behind and the bond linking them to the parents is threatened. Important role models disappear, and family supervision/discipline may be weakened if "parental" authority is not wisely delegated. The second option, taking the children to the destination country, generates other challenges: for example, finding help with child care in the absence of an extended family. Language differences between the two countries also pose a problem. The second generation may not be able to communicate fluently in the mother tongue used by the rest of the relatives, thus weakening the ties and further isolating them from family and community activities.

Traveling with spouses presents a new set of concerns. The nurse's husband—or less frequently, wife—may not be granted a work permit or may not find employment. If a wife works and a husband does not, or if a wife has a better job than her husband, the traditional balance of power between spouses no longer exists. Some advocates of more egalitarian relationships between the sexes would argue that this is a positive step, but it is one that is often difficult to accept, given cultural and societal norms. Not all couples negotiate the change successfully.

Additional problems arise when one spouse wants to return to their native country and another does not. Several nurses who immigrated with their families mentioned that it was their husband who decided when they would return to the homeland. Although these women would have preferred to stay in their new country, they were obliged to follow their husbands.

If a nurse brings her children with her, she has to help them adjust to a new environment, and sometimes she sees them become unfamiliar citizens of an alien culture. Different and sometimes conflicting value systems between the destination and source countries may exacerbate the normal tensions between parents and children.

Yet in other cases, migrant nurses face separation from their children when they return home and the children decide to stay in the adopted destination country. As the world's populations age, dependence on the children for care of the elderly is likely to happen more often and occupy more time. Mobile and separated families will have to deal with these physical and psychological needs as best they can. An indirect consequence for the home country is the loss of the knowledge and skills that could have been contributed by later generations of this family.

And finally, separation from the family and ethnic communities may reduce access to suitable marriage partners if religious or ethnic limitations are strictly imposed. On the other hand, transcultural marriages may be promoted, changing the nature of future national populations.

Reconstructing social networks is no easy task. Most people build their social networks with persons met at the workplace. Colleagues in their new country may or may not welcome migrant nurses. As debates about the nursing shortage escalate in different countries and recruitment bonuses multiply, many homegrown nurses begin to feel that migrants are being given special privileges inaccessible to them and that the presence of migrants allows the health system to ignore the need to retain veteran nursing staff. This can create not only a political and professional wedge between colleagues but a social one as well.

Denise Duvoisin is not alone when she recounts that colleagues in her first job abroad treated her as a second-class professional and completely ignored her socially. The acute loneliness she experienced was hard to accept and extremely demoralizing. Yet, nurses who are invited to socialize with colleagues may find it hard to adjust to cultural differences and expectations. If your religion forbids you to drink, smoke, or dance, how do you adapt to a culture in which all those activities are not only common but expected? And the reverse is also true. How do nurses change basic patterns of social interaction and still integrate their new milieu? Many migrants thus establish their own cultural enclaves that allow them to socialize in familiar ways, but this may create further feelings of estrangement. That the difficult and sometimes tragic stories of migrants fill the pages of so many novels and inspire the plots of countless movies is testament to the enduring problems migrants face worldwide.

Discrimination

Perhaps the most serious problem migrant nurses encounter is racism and discrimination. While discrimination against migrant nurses violates the basic principles represented and articulated by health systems and their personnel, it exists throughout the sector. Migrant nurses are frequent victims of poorly enforced equal-opportunity policies and pervasive double standards. To determine how frequently this occurs is difficult since incidents are often hidden by a blanket of silence and are rarely openly acknowledged.[13]

The sad reality is that some migrant nurses endure nightmarish situations where colleagues purposefully pretend to misunderstand them, try to undermine their professional skills, refuse to help them, and sometimes even bully them, all of which increases the nurses' sense of isolation. The link between discrimination and bullying is clear in many cases and highly destructive, not only to the direct victim but for all those who witness the abuse. Alice Winston*, a Jamaican nurse, remembers that what made her culture shock so intense was the prevalent racism in her hospital in the United States—racism that came, interestingly, not only from native-born nurses

but from other migrant groups. "There was bias in the assignments and ros-
tering. Colleagues would set me up to make mistakes. They would leave out
vital information in the reports between shifts. The Filipino nurses would
talk together in their language. They created a clique—I felt marginalized,
an outcast. The other nurses intimidated me. Racism is scary. You get attacked because of your ethnic origins. It's hard to accept. I finally had to get
the supervisor to intervene and the problem was solved. A great deal depends on the attitude taken by management."

De-skilling—the loss of skills due to lack of regular practice or active
use—is often a serious concern to migrant nurses and constitutes a type of
discrimination that is both an emotional and professional insult. "Although
I had a surgical background, they assigned me to a psychiatric ward," Winston explains. "The Filipino nurses were said to be afraid of big male mental patients and refused to work there. Jamaican nurses were therefore
routinely assigned to these wards regardless of their experience and skills.
Many of the Jamaican nurses left because this was not their area." Among
the ones that stayed, de-skilling and "brain waste" were common, as their
particular nursing expertise was not utilized.

This lack of regard for past expertise negates nurses' sense of professional
worth, undermines their confidence,[14] and contributes to the deterioration
of a much-needed skill pool. The world's population, with its ever-increas-
ing health care needs, cannot afford to be deprived of valuable knowledge
and clinical expertise, and yet the practice is widespread.

Conventional wisdom would have us believe that discrimination occurs
primarily in situations where wide cultural or race differences are involved.
But this was not what Ann Baird*, an English nurse, found when she migrated to Australia, a primarily Caucasian country she originally did not
consider foreign. "I thought it would be like England only with more sun. I
was very unpleasantly surprised by the open hostility to everything English.
This began on my first meeting with the matron, who denied all knowledge
of my arrangements to undertake midwifery training. This despite the letter I showed her that she had written to me. She made it very clear that she
did not like English people. There was no real support during the initial difficult time, but I guess I grew up and got on with it."

According to Per Godtland Kristensen, international secretary of the Norwegian Nurses Association, discrimination in promotion and continuing education opportunities for nurses originating from foreign cultures (Asia and
Africa in particular) was revealed through research commissioned in 2001
by the association. More surprising, are the claims of harassment recently
filed by a group of Finnish nurses working in the north of Norway.

The Nordic countries each have their own culture, language, and traditions. The Finnish language is entirely different from Norwegian, while Swedish and Danish are close enough to facilitate easy communication. In all Nordic countries, however, there are many common legislated structures and procedures as well as the mutual recognition of nursing qualifications. Cultural disorientation and necessary adaptation would be expected to be minimal in the case of these migrant nurses. The Finnish nurses, however, felt themselves harassed and discriminated against. Their speaking Norwegian with an accent and less fluency—an insignificant difference between nationals and non-nationals—was blamed for the abusive practices. Fortunately, in this case, as soon as the issue was raised, strategies were put in place to eliminate the injustice. Many migrant nurses feel that even within very egalitarian societies, they are treated as second-class citizens and, regardless of how well they speak, continue to be treated as strangers.[15]

Even within the Commonwealth countries, different English accents can provoke hurtful laughter, ridicule, and exclusion. Like Ann Baird, Chris Spencer moved from one Commonwealth country to another—from New Zealand to Australia. "One thing that was hard to get used to was having my New Zealand accent made fun of almost daily," she recalls. "You'd think that with so many Kiwis living in Queensland they'd be used to our accents by now, but no!"[16]

Recent Australian research documents that migrant nurses are often treated differently on the basis of their language background.[17] Analyzing the career paths of English-speaking background (ESB) and non-English-speaking background (NESB) migrant nurses, Lesleyanne Hawthorne concluded that discrimination is indisputable. While both ESB and NESB nurses secured professional employment once they had gained registration, significant and persistent labor market segmentation was evident over time. NESB nurses proved to be much less likely than ESB nurses to have progressed beyond baseline registered nursing employment or achieved more than minimal access to higher managerial or nurse supervisor positions, this despite their appropriate qualifications and relative seniority. Furthermore, NESB nurses, especially East Europeans and non-Commonwealth Asian nurses, were disproportionately concentrated in the stigmatized geriatric care sector.

Hawthorne's study reports that discrimination may also target specific groups of migrant nurses. Many NESB nurses spontaneously reported serious and discomforting levels of Australian nurse peer rejection.[18]

A Filipino nurse believed rejection resulted from "only my color and the way I pronounced words (so) that you are always laughed at, degraded." Middle Eastern nurses outlined "hidden and clear discrimination" as well as outright "racism by Anglo-Saxon nurses." . . . An Indonesian nurse perceived her nursing skills to be compromised by exclusion from teams. . . . A Czech nurse said, "I remained always a foreigner not accepted among Australian colleagues" . . . while another described being the constant target of "discrimination and prejudice and backstabbing" from colleagues and administration.[19]

One migrant nurse in the United Kingdom, originally from Zambia, remarks: "I think you are made to realize what color you are, something that you never thought about at home."[20] Any difference appears to be fair game when discriminatory practices are permitted.

In the *American Journal of Nursing*, Michele A. Baqi-Aziz, a Muslim nurse practitioner in the United States, wrote about the discrimination she endured at the hands of other nurses when she wears the *khimar*, the head covering many Muslim women wear. In response to several letters from readers, the editor-in-chief of the journal observed that the profession needs to acknowledge that some nurses are biased against or simply ignorant of the diverse cultures and religions that make up the United States.[21] Another editorial comment pointed out that "as long as Ms. Baqi-Aziz proclaims her religion by wearing *khimar*, she will probably continue to experience prejudice, because she looks different from the norm. There may be some comfort, however, in the fact that, as time goes by, the norm will likely change."[22] This is, of course, poor consolation for those experiencing discrimination now.

In some countries, discrimination targets racial and ethnic minority citizens in the country regardless of migrant status. In the 2003 survey of Royal College of Nursing members, black and ethnic minority nurses were more likely to be working in care homes and older people's nursing than white nurses. A larger proportion of ethnic minority nurses have additional jobs (44 percent compared with 24 percent of white respondents), implying lower basic salaries or greater financial need. Twice as many ethnic minority nurses are taking on the responsibilities of a superior grade but fewer are paid to do so. Ethnic minority nurses are also much less likely to feel that their current grade is appropriate to their role than white nurses (24 percent compared to 50 percent).[23] Finally, one-third of black and ethnic minority nurses report having experienced racial problems with other nurses.

Trevor Philipps, chair of the UK Commission for Racial Equality, claims that the National Health Service is chronically and consistently racially biased in the way it deals with patients and staff.[24] It is not surprising, when permanent staff are subjected to discriminatory practices, that migrant nurses from black and ethnic minority groups are as well. Racial discrimination was more likely to be felt by migrant nurses on lower salaries and those with less experience, suggesting a link between racism and social status.[25]

Less common are affirmative action or positive discrimination policies. For example, when the apartheid regime ended in South Africa, affirmative action was introduced to redress the racial injustices of the past. The policy quickly created new winners and losers. Black students and workers were granted preference within certain quotas. White students and workers as a result had fewer opportunities. As we learned earlier, the South African nurse Mady van de Merve and her two children decided to move to Australia in part because they felt efforts to reverse past discriminatory policies in their homeland had put them at a disadvantage.

Employers, supervisors, and colleagues are not the only ones who discriminate against migrant nurses. The RCN declared that two-thirds of black and ethnic minority nurses report they have experienced racial harassment from patients. In some cases, patients have refused care given by nurses from certain ethnic groups or nationalities. Such behavior is not unique to the United Kingdom. In her unit Denise Duvoisin had several Swiss patients who totally rejected a German nurse because of their forty-year-old memories of World War II. Discrimination is pervasive and may be practiced by a wide range of groups, some quite unexpected.

For decades, the pay and benefits of foreign nurses contracted to work in the Middle East depended on where they had been educated. Although employed as professional nurses under the same working conditions, those coming from the more industrialized countries, like the United States, the United Kingdom, and Australia, were paid higher salaries than those emigrating from the Philippines, China, or India. This was the generalized practice, which went for the most part unchallenged by the nurses from developing countries, who accepted the lower pay as an inevitable characteristic of employment.

New sources of discrimination are constantly emerging. African nurses hired in the United Kingdom were suddenly singled out and stigmatized when some of their colleagues were found to be HIV positive. The barrage of media articles and public pressure on the British health authorities compelled the government to consider reviewing testing procedures on nurses from overseas—screening foreign nurses for HIV/AIDS before allowing them to work in the United Kingdom. When the press painted Africa as the source of the AIDS pandemic and African nurses as a potential threat to the United Kingdom population, a difficult situation was created for these nurses. It is still unclear if the government intends to introduce the additional screening policy, and whether a positive test would disqualify a nurse or a physician from working in the British NHS.[26] According to an RCN legal adviser, "the screening of overseas nurses for HIV and Hepatitis B and C before they are recruited could be construed as unlawful discrimination."[27]

Similarly, during the 2002–3 epidemic of severe acute respiratory syndrome (SARS), many Filipino workers felt they were being victimized and discriminated against. Support groups defending the Filipino workers claimed that the fear of SARS was used to validate discrimination and racism against Filipinos and other Asians. Cecilia Diocson of the Filipino Nurses Support Group in Canada expressed concern when Canadian employers refused to interview some Filipino applicants. "We are already among Canada's low-wage earners. With SARS, our marginalization and exploitation are intensified," she said.[28]

The motivation behind discriminatory practices is not always straightforward and obvious. While it may sometimes be generated by outright racial, ethnic, or religious prejudice, other factors may come into play. At times, foreign nurses may interpret actions as racist or bigoted when in fact they are the result of a more complex set of dilemmas completely independent of their ethnic background. Today, many homegrown nurses feel that employers are exercising a kind of reverse discrimination in their dealings with loyal staff. They see hospitals and health care institutions wooing new recruits with sign-on bonuses, housing and travel subsidies, educational subsidies, and promises of good schedules unavailable to them. Nurses struggling with the daily realities of the workplace—low salaries, poor working conditions, high workloads, and few acceptable accommodation options—are amazed that the same efforts made to help migrant nurses settle are not routinely extended to them. National nurses may sometimes perceive the support given to the internationally recruited nurses as preferential treatment and a form of discrimination against them.[29]

Orientation, free on-site training, and facilitated further education are advantages that all nurses would like to receive but presently seem to be reserved for migrant nurses. Jealousies of this nature will not nurture acceptance, integration, and team building. Nurses in Northern Ireland, for example, recently expressed concern when a local trust recruited twenty-five nurses from the Philippines on two-year contracts while they were being kept on short-term contracts. They wanted assurances that foreign nurses were not being given preference when applying for permanent hospital posts.[30]

In many industrialized countries suddenly plagued by a shortage of nurses, internationally recruited staff may be welcomed initially. If these first experiences in immigration are successful, health systems often decide to incorporate even more foreign nurses into the workforce. Some reservations begin to be expressed, however, when the numbers dramatically increase, especially in countries where workforces traditionally share a similar culture and language. In such cases, nurses already working in the units are asked to orient the migrant nurses and incorporate them into the work life. This means increased pressure and workload for nurses already stressed because of the staff shortage. The potential culture clash and rising resentment may lead nurses to be less than welcoming to their new colleagues. Whatever discrimination these migrant nurses experience, however, arises as much from system problems as from cultural or ethnic prejudice.

The reality is that if migrant nurses are badly treated, they may choose to move again, to return home or settle in yet another country. Indeed, the fact that they have migrated once makes a second move all the more likely.

The Kurdish nurse Fatima Ansari, whom we met in chapter 1, surmounted many of the challenges described above. She faced discrimination at home and also abroad. When Ansari was in Sweden, she consulted an employment agency and was reassured that whatever she wanted on the labor market was accessible. Her only obstacle was language. She enrolled in an intensive language course to learn Swedish, but even with that hurdle negotiated, she was to encounter more.

The employment agency arranged for her knowledge test and an exam on health regulations in Sweden. "Every test was a nightmare," Ansari recalls. "I managed to get my Swedish qualifications in three years—it usually takes much longer, up to six years. In the meantime, I worked as a nursing assistant, which did not require nursing qualifications."

Although Ansari had to deal with loneliness, made more acute by the dark Swedish winter nights, she sometimes found the stark contrast between Sweden and the Middle East strangely reassuring. She was finally very far away from the oppressive conditions that led her to migrate. "I felt very safe among my new colleagues—more than in my native country. My sister and brother (not nurses) have very different perspectives. My brother, who was trained in information technology, could not find a job in his profession and is now a bus driver. My sister has a degree in political science and has not been able to find employment. She is very, very bitter. Nursing gives me better opportunities. I have the right job and the right education. I am a foreigner in Sweden but this I can accept. I could not accept being treated as a foreigner in my own country."

"I worked eleven years in my home country and was very unhappy," she continued. "I am now in Sweden and I am happy. I can plan my life. I wish to specialize in critical care and disaster relief. I know I can do that here. I dream of going to Africa and working in humanitarian aid. It wasn't easy leaving everything familiar to me, but I feel very lucky."

This courageous and determined woman closed the interview by saying, "Thank you for listening to my story—no one has asked me to tell it before." Stories such as hers are critical. They need to be heard and must inform migration and labor policy in source and destination countries.

3. Mini-Business, Big Business

When she graduated nursing school Jane Benito[†] was twenty-two years old. She had lived in Button City all her life and was the fifth of seven children. Her parents were poor and struggled to make ends meet. But they paid the US$4,000–$7,000 for the four-year program given by a private for-profit nursing school in the Philippines. Its curriculum was specifically designed to provide Jane with the education and skills she would need to provide economic support to her family and, at the same time, to migrate.

When she looked for employment after graduation, there were no decent jobs to be found at home. Two of her uncles had already migrated to the United States, and they encouraged her to hunt for a job there. All she had to do was open the daily newspaper, and there the jobs were—ads for hospitals all over the world as well as ads for recruitment agencies that would serve as intermediaries between Filipino nurses and health care facilities looking for staff.

Benito decided to go the recruitment agency route and was lucky enough to find one that would not steal her money and renege on its promises. They put her into contact with an employer in Texas who started the procedures for her work permit. The agency then helped her take the professional pre-licensure exam (developed and administered by CGFNS). When she passed it, they advanced her the money to travel to Texas to take the US licensing exam (NCLEX-RN) and provided free accommodation for her first month in the United States. With her first paycheck, she began to pay her family back—and reimburse the recruitment agency for the money advanced to cover expenses.

[†] A dagger symbol indicates a fictitious composite interviewee.

Nurses like Jane Benito are following an increasingly common career trajectory. For them, finding a good job often means jumping on the migration superhighway until they reach the employment destination of their choice. Some nurses have a relatively easy time, some do not. But for all, the highway is littered with obstacles. To negotiate each one requires services from people or institutions that usually demand something in return. As in Benito's case, their first step on the journey involves an educational institution. Next, they have to find out about a job. This means looking for ads in nursing journals or newspapers or on the web, or engaging the services of an international or local employment recruiter. Nurses have to make sure they have the right credentials and licensing, which might mean taking a certain number of exams to meet the requirements of the country chosen as a final destination. Finally, they need to apply for the right visa and pay the necessary fees. For some nurses, a lawyer might be needed. There are innumerable roadblocks to negotiate, their passage made more difficult if nurses are not adequately informed or are deliberately misinformed.

When workers move across a border, a continent, or an ocean, there are usually multiple middlemen or organizations involved in that journey. These businessmen or organizations first appear when only a few individuals make the move. When migration exists on a massive scale—as is the case with nurses—the business opportunities are endless. In today's global nursing marketplace, mini-business and big business alike are discovering and exploiting the potential of profit-making ventures. Travel agents, recruiters, lawyers, and advertising agencies are not the only players involved. In countries where there is a large public sector, these nonprofit public health services are increasingly managed as businesses and are on the lookout for private investment initiatives. The public and private health care sectors together are the biggest employer in most countries. This labor-intensive industry depends on and generates a massive parallel and interlinking chain of enterprises, each one claiming to contribute to the delivery of health care services.

Trade in services cannot exist without individuals providing the services. Because nursing is the largest occupational category in health care, nurses play a pivotal role in the trade of health services. Since international nurse recruitment has become one of the quickest ways to get nurses to the sites where there are dire shortages of health services, people are willing to pay anyone who can facilitate migration. Increased international recruitment has strengthened preexisting businesses, encouraged expansions or international partnerships, and stimulated the creation of many new small and medium-size enterprises.

"Migration streams, seen as mobility streams, are dynamic and pliant, involve different types of people and motivations, have different roles and methods of insertion into host societies, and are influenced and managed by different agencies and institutions," reports John Salt of the University College of London. "They present, and result from, wide-ranging business opportunities. . . . Today, international migration can also be regarded as a diverse international business, with a vast budget, providing hundreds of thousands of jobs worldwide and managed by a set of individuals, agencies and institutions, each of which has an interest in developing a sector of the business."[1] Or as, Debi Gamble puts it, "It takes a village to successfully coordinate and integrate the multiple and parallel processes involved."[2]

To direct traffic in the global village, a number of intermediary institutions and enterprises manage the stream of migrants, including migrant nurses. For the individual attracted to nursing and planning to practice the profession in a foreign country, the road may be long and circuitous, dotted with a seemingly endless variety of "tollbooths." As nurses pass through them, hands stretch out demanding a fee. To understand nurse migration, therefore, we have to look at the various institutional and entrepreneurial actors that have erected these tollbooths. What motivates this business growth and where is the financial gain? What are the benefits and costs to countries, health systems, nurses, and patients? What is the potential for exploitation in this new global marketplace with its myriad new business opportunities? How does business in the new global health care village shape and interact with other social institutions?

Step One: Getting an Education

Although the educational sector in most countries has numerous ties to business—and certainly prepares people for the workplace—education is not usually viewed as a major marketplace activity. But in the world of skilled workers who circumnavigate the globe, educational institutions have become key actors and are engaged in a complex interplay with the business community. As more and more business ties are forged, clear boundaries between scholarship—or even vocational training—and commerce blur. Educational institutions do not just impart the skills and knowledge necessary for workers to move into business or service institutions in the national economy. They are increasingly and deliberately viewing themselves as a kind of intellectual manufacturing sector, one of whose missions is to produce workers for the global labor market. Indeed, some colleges and universities have become high-end technical schools that are fashioning their future worker products for export to particular markets, tailoring their courses and skills to suit a special market niche. In an even closer tie with the market they service, many state-run educational institutions are forging partnerships with government allowing both parties to solve different sets of social, political, or economic challenges. What is more, a number of for-profit educational enterprises that are not connected to universities have entered the lucrative business niche of servicing the international market as opposed to the domestic one. Finally, even recruitment agencies are playing a new and surprising role in the educational market by creating connections to educational institutions that give them an edge in the competition.

All of this is possible, of course, because education is the absolute foundation of the globalization of skilled professionals like nurses. No nurse can move either internally or externally if she does not have the proper education. A wide selection of institutions, courses, and programs are available, at times custom-made to fit market needs.

The fate and direction of nursing education, like all other areas of higher education, is intimately connected to political and social decisions. Financial decisions have a major impact on nursing programs, whether the program depends on public funding or is highly privatized. In the 1980s and 1990s, both governments and the health industry initiated financial constraints and budget cuts that had a significant impact on the schools that educate nurses. Hospitals laid off nurses, and governments closed many publicly funded nursing schools. They decreased faculty positions and reduced the student enrollment. These cost-containment measures were not restricted to the developing world—countries like Trinidad and Tobago.[3] Canada and the United Kingdom also deliberately reduced the inflow of nurses to the labor market. Even in the largely for-profit US health care system with its many privately financed nursing schools, cuts in nursing staff resulted in fewer school applicants, smaller student bodies, the closure of schools, and the layoff of faculty. Many believe that these policies are partly responsible for the dramatic nurse shortage experienced today.

A growing number of industrialized countries like the United States, the United Kingdom, and Australia have recently reversed these trends, increasing health-sector budget allocations in order to finance more student places and offer additional educational scholarships. This will have an immediate impact on educational facilities whose revenues will increase and whose programs and activities may expand. Even with this expansion, the number of nurses produced cannot hope to compensate anytime soon for the numbers that have been lost because of previous fiscal tightening and restructuring. Both commercial and government actors in a variety of different countries are thus poised to help fill the gaps. For them, the production of nurses for export has multiple benefits.

Government-run and even private educational institutions are well paid for their partnerships with foreign institutions in the production process, thus contributing to the economic growth of the country. In addition, governments faced with large numbers of unemployed workers are able to reduce the burden on social welfare programs, but more importantly, they can reliably count on money being sent home by the migrant workers to their families, improving the general standard of living of the population.

There is no better example of how this dynamic works than China, which has made significant business investments in the training of workers for export. This new move is a consequence of the government's 1996 decision to lay off nine million public-sector workers. To address the resulting social crisis, the government has strongly encouraged emigration. Across China the government has set up 160 training facilities that are specifically designed to make citizens more attractive to foreign employers. This has already facilitated employment abroad for 140,000 people—some of them nurses.[4] While these efforts do not specifically target nurses, the government understands the potential of nurses as a product for overseas export. To support employment abroad, the Chinese government has created scholarships and negotiated government-to-government labor agreements. The message is clear: Chinese nurses face a wider range of job prospects abroad than they do at home.

Industrialized countries consider the 1.2 million Chinese nurses an untapped and almost inexhaustible reservoir of staff. Countries like Saudi Arabia, the United States, the United Kingdom, Ireland, and Australia, to name only a few, have already recruited Chinese nurses. And educational institutions in many of them are implementing programs that allow them to exploit this huge market. At Curtin University in Western Australia, conversion courses have been designed to allow foreign-educated nurses (among them Chinese students) to obtain internationally recognized degrees that facilitate entry to the international labor market. Both the Chinese and Australians benefit. The Chinese effectively retrain and manage their surplus labor, and Curtin gets paid handsomely for each foreign student. Needless to say, the university benefits greatly if more foreign nurses take advantage of these programs.

Many other exchange and collaborative student and faculty programs have been formed between Chinese universities and institutions abroad. These include universities in Asia, the South Pacific, and North America. The aim of these programs is to upgrade Chinese nursing education. Inevitably this will also facilitate international recognition of their qualifica-tions or competencies (knowledge and skills) and thus promote migration. Needless to say, it is also extremely lucrative for educational institutions in the countries that train foreign nurses, especially when fees for foreign stu-dents are significantly higher than the fees charged national or long-term resident students.

On November 21, 2002, the Chinese official Xinhua news agency an-nounced the agreement for a new US CGFNS test center in Beijing. Accord-ing to the commission's website, the CGFNS certification program is

> designed specifically for first-level general nurses educated and licensed out-side the United States who wish to assess their chances of passing the US registered nurse licensing exam, the NCLEX-RN examination, and attaining licensure to practice as registered nurses within the United States. The pro-gram is comprised of three parts: a credential review of the nurse's educa-tion, registration and licensure; the CGFNS Qualifying Exam, a one-day qualifying exam testing nursing knowledge; and an English language profi-ciency exam. Upon successful completion of all three elements of the pro-gram, the applicant is awarded a CGFNS Certificate.

Again according to CGFNS, "a CGFNS Certificate helps applicants [to] meet state requirements for the registered nurse licensure exam [and] qualify for an occupational visa."[5]

This decision on the part of the Chinese government to establish a test center in Beijing implicitly facilitates the migration of Chinese nurses to the United States and produces "a stimulus for further integration of China, in-cluding Chinese nursing, into the global community."[6] According to Piyasiri Wickramasekara of the International Migration Programme of the Interna-tional Labour Office, China was not, until recently, unduly concerned with what is called the "brain drain"—the negative impact of the loss of masses of skilled workers. On the contrary, it viewed the stock of Chinese skilled workers overseas as a "brain bank," or "brain power stored abroad."

Indeed, in a strange twist to the story, direct access to CGFNS is thought to be the last chance of survival for the five hundred diploma schools (edu-cational programs run by hospitals rather than community colleges or uni-versities) left in China. "Rural communities with vastly unfilled needs present little appeal to nurses. On the other hand, urban hospitals that have attracted nurses traditionally have difficulties hiring more nurses due to the so-called 'staffing quota formula' (*ding bian*), which privileges medical and administrative personnel over nurses," Yu Xu reports. In addition, "most ur-ban hospitals have shifted to a hiring policy of favoring graduates of asso-ciate and baccalaureate nursing programs as a measure to improve nursing care quality, leaving graduates of secondary nursing schools even smaller survival space."[7]

Policy changes adopted by the United States and China may have different motivating factors and distinct impacts in each country. What is obvious is that interdependence exists in a globalized world. In fact, change introduced in two countries often influences developments in other parts of the world. For example, if masses of Chinese nurses migrate to the United States, other countries suffering from shortages may not be able to fill their vacancies. So countries like Ireland, the United Kingdom, and Australia will have to spend more time developing ties with other countries to satisfy their demand for migrant nurses. Creative solutions will bring about change and the nurse recruitment process will once again evolve, implicating perhaps new potential source countries or more energetic efforts to recruit and retain domestically educated nurses.

China is only one of the many countries in which either government or business actors have exploited the labor and commercial opportunities created by the international demand and migration of nurses. In spite of the critical nursing shortage, governments in some developing countries are continuing to cut back the budget for training and reduce the number of educational institutions for nurses. That does not necessarily mean that nursing education is drastically cut because, in a number of countries, for-profit private-sector companies are opening up their own nursing schools. This is true of South Africa, where "private hospitals have picked up much of the slack" and are training thousands of nurses.[8] The profitable business of establishing and marketing private schools of nursing is perhaps nowhere as prevalent as in the Philippines. In the 1970s there were 63 schools of nursing, and by 1998 this number had increased to 198.[9] In 2004 this number had nearly doubled, with 370 nursing programs in the country—most of them private. The growing concern is that the regulatory process does not have adequate inspection mechanisms and human resources to apply them. At the same time, private companies may charge exorbitant prices, forcing students into heavy debt. This in turn often obliges them to find better-paying jobs abroad once they graduate in order to pay back their loans.

"Despite our Herculean efforts to stop the opening of more and more colleges and schools, we are helpless because the hospitals that open these schools are owned by doctors, who as a group are very strong and powerful," explains the dean of the University of the Philippines College of Nursing, Leonor Malay Aragon. Nursing, she says

> has become one of the most expensive careers for girls to take and a most profitable one for the hospital owners. Where girls in this country were paid

before to take up Nursing and given all kinds of inducements like free board and lodging, they now pay huge sums—to the hospitals for affiliation fees, books, board and lodging. Indeed, the possibilities of making money through a nursing school is limitless. And the free service that students render to patients while learning is not even given value in the final cost of accounting. Since they spend so much for their education, naturally their tendency after graduation is to go abroad.[10]

New business opportunities in nursing education also abound because more and more health care facilities are creating partnerships with schools of nursing. Although such partnerships are often hailed as new and innovative, they are in fact, decades, even centuries, old. Ever since nursing was professionalized in the nineteenth century, nurses have been educated in schools that were run by hospitals. Nursing students provided cheap labor for these hospitals while they were studying, and some of them remained in full employment when they graduated. Until the mid-twentieth century, the hospital school, which usually awarded its graduates a "diploma" after three years of study and clinical training, was the primary educator of most nurses worldwide. These programs established a direct link between service and training. The advancement of nursing science, however, imposed changes in the education formula, putting greater emphasis on theory and scientific knowledge.

When nursing education entered universities and became a responsibility of the Ministry of Education or university faculty and administrators, a split between service and education could be seen. Interestingly, the new business of nursing education may be reducing this division as hospitals and other health care facilities become close-knit partners once again, both directly involved in nursing education. In an effort to ensure sufficient nurses for their services, health care facilities are now establishing partnerships with universities and training institutions, helping financially to accommodate both student and faculty needs.

One example of this is a program that has been pioneered by several community health care facilities and Boise State University. According to the American Association of Colleges of Nursing, "Boise State University was able to expand capacity with financial assistance from community health care facilities and through targeted marketing efforts aimed at both students and faculty."[11]

Innovative programs with more flexible workplace-based courses are being offered at Regis University in Colorado. "We have developed partnerships with Health One and the University of Colorado Hospital to offer an on-site Bachelor of Science in Nursing (BSN) program for their employees, which has been very well received," said nursing program director Candace

Berardinelli.[12] While these initiatives are not producing nurses for export, they are an attempt to reduce the demand for imported nurses.

These health care and education partnerships also exist in developing countries. Fortune Medicare (Philippines) is exploring the possibility of establishing its own nursing school or linking with a university in order to ensure easier access to nursing staff for their fifteen clinics. And in South Africa, Netcare (Network Healthcare Holdings) runs five nursing schools throughout the country with two thousand entry-level nurses actually in training. According to Dr. Richard Friedland, chief operating officer,

> the Netcare group, the largest integrated private healthcare organization in southern Africa, owns and manages 45 hospitals comprising 7,200 beds, 319 operating theatres, 61 specialized medical centers and is supported by 2,200 medical specialists. The group also owns and manages 53 Medicross Family Medical and Dental Centres. Collectively, medical facilities within the Netcare group care for over 4.8 million patients a year. . . . Netcare International is a division that is dedicated to expanding the group's involvement in the international healthcare arena. The Netcare group employs 18,000 staff and generated R3.6 billion (US$573 million) turnover for the financial year ending September 2001.[13]

Once again, the domestic production of much-needed nurses has encouraged partnerships between the health care providers (even international commercial chains) and educational institutions. That link is sometimes so tight that new schools are established directly under the umbrella of the provider enterprise. The advantage to the health care facility is having cheap labor during the years of study and the opportunity to establish a relationship that may become an employment contract once the student graduates. Schools may offer their nursing education programs free of financial burden but instead require that new graduates pay back the cost of their education by working a determined number of years. The duration may be anything from a single year up to the total number of years (three or four) of the nurse's education. This process is known as "bonding" students. In the case of Netcare with its international provider contracts, nurses may stay employed by the chain and yet work abroad, outside of South Africa.

Education becomes part of the business venture in another way. One very significant perk or benefit that encourages nurses to migrate is the promise of enhanced or advanced education. Hospitals offer nurses educational stipends or promise to pay for their education if a nurse decides to go back to school or enroll in a course that will certify her for a new or needed area of practice. Thus, if Nurse Fontaine[†] has worked as a medical surgical nurse but wants to become an oncology nurse, her hospital may pay for her to take a course to get a special certification. Or, if she has a two-year community college degree or a three-year degree, it may be in the interest of the hospital to pay for the "bridge course" to get her higher university education, a BSN, and perhaps a master's or doctorate.

Educational stipends are of enormous mutual benefit. Hospitals can use the promise of these benefits to gain a competitive edge in the employment marketplace while upgrading the skills and education level of its staff. This is particularly useful since it gives the institution a better-educated nurse with greater loyalty to the institution that has helped nurture her personal and professional development. Scholarships of this nature continue to significantly contribute to the enhancement of nursing knowledge and clinical skills, especially in developing countries with limited educational opportunities. Stipends are also very important to educational institutions, particularly when state funds are limited.

These kinds of perks have typically been used in internal markets and they are becoming ever more important in the global search for skilled nurses. Thus, one of the lures that US hospital recruiters use when they go to Canada is the promise that their employer will give nurses educational stipends that many Canadian hospitals eliminated during the cost cutting of the 1990s.

Employer/university partnerships are also targeting new student populations to expand their income base as well as increase the numbers of nurse graduates for hire. As seen earlier, in 2004 approximately four thousand physicians in the Philippines were taking accelerated courses to become nurses. This unprecedented phenomenon affirms the high market value of nurses, particularly in the international labor market. "Now, it seems the most sought-after person in a hospital isn't the doctor. It is the registered nurse."[14]

Similar projects have begun in the United States. A private-sector partnership between Hospital Corporation of America, Mercy, Cedars and Kendall Regional Medical Center, and Florida International University (FIU) created the Physicians-to-Nursing program. In December 2003, thirty-two foreign physicians from Cuba, Romania, Haiti, Nicaragua, Mexico, the Dominican Republic, and the Philippines graduated with nursing degrees after a three-semester course with weekend clinical rotations.[15] Like Jean Fenelon, introduced in chapter 2, these physicians were residing in the United States but were unable to practice medicine.

Australian and German nursing schools are also training physicians to be nurses. Stephen Van Vorst, director of undergraduate studies in the Faculty of Nursing, Midwifery and Health of the University of Technology in Sydney, says that each year the school enrolls a handful of physicians from other countries, particularly China. The students' qualifications in medicine (most commonly traditional Chinese medicine) have not been recognized in Australia, and they are unable to obtain registration as a physician. "Because the department of immigration lists nursing as an area of high demand, it is much easier to get study or work in Australia for nursing students and professionals." Labor market demand and professional practice standards will determine if this type of retraining program will continue.

Foundations have financially supported the creation of special university programs targeting foreign-educated health professionals to facilitate their reentry into active practice. Colleges in San Francisco and Los Angeles received $4 million in funding from the California Endowment Foundation to help foreign-trained health professionals qualify to work in the United States. Initially, this program expects to help an estimated twelve hundred California residents who originally trained as health professionals in more than seventy-five countries, and the number is expected to grow.[16]

Increasingly, health-sector stakeholders—ministries or departments of health, health care facilities, consumer groups (including parliamentarians or members of Congress), insurers, and commercial enterprises like pharmaceutical companies—are providing scholarships in order to encourage graduates and mature students to enter nursing. It is not unusual for governments, health care facilities, or educational institutions to provide impressive incentives. For example, Tenet Healthcare Foundation, a philanthropic arm of Tenet Healthcare Corporation, awarded a $1 million grant to the East Los Angeles Community Union Education Foundation to provide financial support to Latino nursing students enrolled in local colleges in 2002.[17] The four-year grant covers tuition, licensing and exam fees, and a stipend for living expenses, computers, and books. While the nurses and hospitals benefit directly from this grant, it is clear that many other institutions and enterprises do as well—for example, universities, suppliers (books, computers), and licensing agencies. These kinds of programs may provide new opportunities for health care professionals who would otherwise be working in jobs outside the health sector, often receiving lower salaries. At the same time, they support local commerce.

On the other hand, the increase in private schools with tuition-based education has in some cases created a financial obstacle for those considering entry into the profession. People genuinely interested in working in nursing are turned away when they cannot pay for their education. There is no doubt that publicly financed nursing schools will continue to be needed if nursing shortages are to be addressed.

What is surprising is the participation of recruitment agencies in education. As we will see later in this chapter, one of the businesses that has both benefited from and fueled nurse migration is the recruitment agency. These agencies are usually for-profit companies that hospitals, other health care facilities, and governments pay to find nurses either at home or abroad. Their expertise is not in education but in employment placements. Because so many new players have entered the recruitment market and the demand for specialized nurses has greatly increased—or because recruitment agencies have been criticized for stealing nurses from poorer countries and selling them to richer ones—recruitment agencies trying to gain a competitive or ethical edge are beginning to venture into the hitherto alien world of education.

It is important to recognize the implications of the new role of recruitment agencies. In the past these agencies simply informed nurses that hospitals might, as an added bonus, provide foreign nurses with educational stipends to upgrade their skills, enter into a new area of practice, or get an advanced degree. Thus the agencies were just passing on information about the benefits that the nurse might find in her new country or institution of employment. Today, however, some recruitment agencies are themselves financing and offering nurses scholarships or establishing educational institutions of their own.

In an attempt to improve its public image as well as attract a bigger share of a lucrative business, for example, one recruitment agency in the Philippines, International Quality Manpower Services, claims that it is concerned with much more than merely recruiting nurses. It offers scholarships that cover full matriculation and incidental expenses; it supports new graduates in securing local licenses to practice, and it obtains local employment for one or two years that will prepare the nurses for eventual placement to the United States. Training courses for foreign licensure are available. In addition, the agency offers grants for master's degree programs to support nurses interested in becoming educators, thus responding to concerns about the falling number of nursing faculty in the Philippines.[18] As the numbers of nurse educators dwindles in the industrialized countries, the international recruitment process has begun to target nurse educators as well as staff nurses. The emigration of nurse educators is seen as a significant business threat for local recruiters, who fear a reduction in student pools.

The Alliance Abroad Group (a US company) is another major recruitment agency that seeks nurses worldwide. "It's all about your life, your dreams. It's all about capturing opportunities, making good choices," their website tells the foreign nurse. To help nurses make these choices and exploit these opportunities, the company has created a subsidiary called Blu-Chip. In response to the severe nursing shortage in the United States, Blu-Chip works with nursing schools and ministries of health in countries like Grenada and Barbados where it recruits. It offers scholarships in the source countries to help prepare nurses, who in return commit themselves for three years to the health care facility that sponsors them.[19] The agency creates the link between health facilities looking for nurses, nurses eager to enter nursing school, ministries of health that support the training of nurses, and schools keen on receiving tuition fees in hard currency. Nurse Howard[†] could therefore benefit from a full scholarship, obtain her nursing diploma, and be licensed to practice in exchange for three years of employment abroad in the profession of her choice. Once these three years are over, Nurse Howard may return to her Caribbean island fully equipped to work in any health care facility, stay on in the United States if her work permit allows, or accept short- or long-term contracts in the United States alternating with time spent in her home country.

Recruitment agencies are also getting directly involved in financing specialty training schools abroad. According to a recent news article, Blue Cross Healthcare in the United Kingdom has established a six-month mental health care conversion course in Kerala, India, which will train general nurses to work in British mental hospitals or community health centers. Public-sector hospitals send representatives to India to screen candidates found by the recruitment agencies. They pay the agency recruitment fee and fund the nurses' entire training. Local tutors and visiting UK lecturers teach the recruits in the school set up in Kerala. The cost to the hospitals is considerably less than the £35,000 currently spent on each nurse taking a UK-based conversion course. Although recruits do not pay for their training, they are expected to sign a three-year contract with the sponsoring facility.[20] No basic, direct-entry mental health training exists in Kerala at present. If the nurses return home after their committed time in the United Kingdom, the training and acquired experience increase the pool of nursing skills in India. This supposes, however, that the Indian health system recognizes the mental health or psychiatric specialty and provides hospitals or other facilities in which to practice the newly acquired skills. The curriculum of such a school would naturally tend to meet the needs, criteria, and standards of (in this case) the United Kingdom, which may be vastly different from local requirements. Preparing nurses for export carries the risk of neglecting national priority health care challenges. On the other hand, the introduction of mental health programs may expand nursing practice in the country and create new career opportunities for the specialist nurse.

Expanding the Education Export Industry

The education export industry is growing at a fast rate because universities are not the only ones to benefit from nurse migration. Governments trying to improve their international balance of payments and forge links with other countries find that they can do this while simultaneously decreasing their subsidies for tertiary education. Industrialized countries face an increasingly critical shortage of skilled labor as their birth rates and numbers of school leavers decrease. Foreign skilled graduates become an excellent pool of workers to draw on. By the time they have finished their foreign study, they are already familiar with the new country's environment and able to integrate easily into the labor market.[21] Worldwide an estimated 1.5 million students are studying overseas.[22] Australia has the second-highest ratio of overseas students (compared to total students) after Switzerland, and the third-highest in absolute numbers after the United States and Britain.[23] A distinction needs to be made between foreign students who have the intention of returning home after graduation and those who plan to stay in the host country. There is no conclusive data, however, to tell us what percentage of foreign students actually do return home.

Matsushima Endo* is typical of students who go abroad only for a short time. Endo's personal dream and professional goal was to care for the elderly. She studied in Japan, obtained her BSN, and started looking for a master's program in gerontological nursing. When she graduated from nursing school, Japan did not have this kind of specialty program, so she decided to go to the United States. There Endo could get the education she needed as well as improve her English. Once she had done both, she returned to Japan, where she practiced her specialty and soon became a nurse educator developing a gerontological nursing curriculum. Active in her professional association, she continues to use her learned language and leadership skills to advance the profession in her country and internationally.

Traditionally, nurses have sought professional development via educational programs that were only accessible abroad. But for many nurses, the educational experience and exposure to new societies profoundly changes their personal goals and life plans. Their intentions to return home may be replaced by the desire to continue their life abroad. Haile Kahsay, whom we met earlier, readily admits that going to the United Kingdom, United States, and Canada to upgrade his nursing qualifications was an opportunity that changed the course of his entire life. "It opened the world for me," he said. Never could he have imagined the life and career possibilities that lay outside his country. The exposure to new customs and behaviors, to a higher standard of living, and to greater professional opportunities convinced Kahsay that his future and that of his family had fundamentally changed. Not everything was better, but he could not return to former ways.

The value of overseas study for nurses and nursing must never be un-

derestimated. It is now clear, however, that overseas students are also critical for the countries offering study and research programs. Taking Australia
as an example, overseas students contributed A$5.2 billion to the economy
in 2002. The growth rate in fee-paying places that year surpassed new places
for domestic students by 3:1. Half of the overseas students in Australia in
2000 were studying in the higher education sector.[24]

Many university administrations, particularly in publicly supported universities, are encouraging the influx of foreign (nonresident) students in a
way that both exploits the commercial potential of out-of-country applicants and fuels nurse migration. While some countries' legislation mandates
equal treatment of national and foreign students, many countries distinguish between them and charge foreigners higher fees for tertiary education
programs. The fees multiplied by a critical mass of students represent a significant amount of money. In some trade agreements, equal treatment of students has been a key issue under negotiation.

Publicly funded Australian universities are currently being pressured by
government to increase their enrollment of foreign students because of the
income-generating potential these students represent. While an Australian
student will pay approximately $3,500 for their government-subsidized
nursing school tuition, a foreign student will pay a minimum of $12,000 and
as much as $18,000. Increasing the number of foreign students thus signifi-
cantly augments the university's revenue. Australia is not the exception.
Take, for example, Louisiana State University in New Orleans. A bachelor's
degree nursing student from out of state pays $850 more than the basic fee
($1,098) charged to state residents. At the master's level the fees are essen-
tially double: $1,261 for a Louisiana student, $2,511 for an out-of-state student. The difference is more dramatic at the London School of Hygiene and
Tropical Medicine, where a master's degree foreign student pays three times
more than the UK citizen or permanent resident. Overseas students have become a major source of survival for academia.

Since 1998, overseas student revenue in Australia has doubled and represents 13 percent of total sector revenue. In some cases, like that of the University of Wollongong or Central Queensland University, overseas students
revenue amounts to 20–38 percent of university funding.[25]

Overseas students also contribute to the general economy. In 2000 they
spent A$1.9 billion on goods and services while in Australia.[26] There is no
doubt that this is big business and a huge market.

Many universities are thus wooing foreign students. Computer technology has enhanced the opportunity to tap into a global market of thousands
of potential students. Courses and degrees are no longer limited to on-site
programs; distance learning options are being offered. Most Australian

nursing schools offer distance learning courses. Taking only one example, academic staff at the School of Nursing Sciences at James Cook University have been working in close partnership with the Ministry of Health and the School of Nursing in Fiji to help meet the education needs of registered nurses there. Faculty from both schools of nursing run transition courses that help the Fijian nurse with a three-year diploma acquire a bachelor's degree via distance education materials, face-to-face teaching at residential schools, and clinical practice.[27]

Distance learning materials require their own teaching methodology. Most often they require computer access and computer skills on the part of both teacher and student. Videotapes also play a central role. These new technologies automatically generate their own cluster of enterprises to support such programs.

Education Industry Support Services

An overview of the education industry cannot be restricted to universities and their on-campus faculty and students. Schools or university departments that teach language skills provide critical support services, since foreign nurses are often asked or required to improve their skills before they can continue studying or get better jobs.

As Australian universities demand language proficiency, the revenue brought by overseas students may not be limited to tertiary-level schools. Robyn Aitken, a doctoral student at the University of Melbourne, for example, has been doing research on Indonesian nurses who participated in a special training program in Australia. In 1999 the Central Java Provincial Ministry of Health offered scholarships to Indonesian teachers of nursing and midwifery to study in Australia as part of the Fifth Health Project, funded by a World Bank loan. This project aimed to improve services to poor and disadvantaged Indonesians. Schools or institutions providing language courses and certification benefited as well. Even though most spoke some English, the candidates needed to improve their language skills, so the teachers traveled to Australia and enrolled in an intensive English course.[28]

Some language schools that benefit from nurse migration operate in the host country, while others are established in the home country. Some are independent of each other; others are branches of a transnational enterprise. For example, La Trobe University in Australia is active in Beijing, where it provides English competency courses to prepare Chinese students for overseas tertiary study.[29]

Consider the Cambridge Certificate of Proficiency in English (CPE), which is well known globally and a prized qualification. It is the highest level of the Cambridge exams in English for Speakers of Other Languages (ESOL). According to the Cambridge ESOL website, the CPE exam is intended "for learners who have achieved a high level of language skills and are able to function effectively in almost any English-speaking context. Every year over 45,000 people take the CPE exam in more than 80 countries, and success at this level represents a significant personal achievement."[30] Acknowledging their clients' need to be guaranteed widespread recognition of this exam, Cambridge makes available a list of the institutions and employers that recognize the CPE certificate—a useful service but also a very good marketing advantage. While the Cambridge exams are perhaps the best known, a multitude of other enterprises, small and large, offer language courses in most every country.

The educational enterprise is producing another layer of entrepreneurial activity. Because students are being recruited from further away, we see the emergence of education agents hired by colleges to recruit students. There are thousands of such agents operating worldwide. In an unregulated environment, anyone can be an education agent—there are no requirements, standards, or codes of conduct. While many education agents serve a legitimate purpose and behave ethically, there have been cases of exploitation. Some commission fees have been abusive—up to 40 percent of the student course fee—and some agents have been involved in immigration scams.[31]

One case came to the attention of Clive Graham of the Australian Council for Private Education and Training. It "involved an agent, an unscrupulous agent overseas, telling parents of Southeast Asian villages that their son or daughter could come to Australia for, say, A$10,000. The poor people in the villages don't have that money, but the agent loans it to them, ostensibly," Graham explains. The agent never actually gives them the money but takes the young person, aged nineteen to twenty-four, to Australia to study English on the pretext that the young person will be able to earn a lot of money in Australia and pay the A$10,000 back, plus A$1,000 commission and another A$10,000 or A$12,000 for the family after just twelve months. "Now when those students have come to Australia," Graham adds, "there is no college for them to attend—they're sleeping four, five, six to a bed, and they have to earn money. In some cases they go and work slave labor in a restaurant, which has been organized for them, and in some cases they're encouraged to enter prostitution." In that way they can earn the A$11,000 to pay the agent, but they will go home empty handed. "We can do nothing about it," Graham concludes, "because the students that were involved fear that their parents will find out, that the authorities will deport them, and they'll be labeled criminals. We have no control because these agents are foreigners, residents of another country."[32]

Many parallels can be drawn with practices of the nurse recruitment agencies we will explore later in this chapter. Once again there is a complete absence of international standards, audit mechanisms, or any severe sanctions for malpractice or fraud. National standards and audits have not been developed and are urgently needed.

Step Two: Getting a Foreign License

Once she is equipped with a recognized diploma or degree, the nurse has only just entered the migration superhighway. To move to her final destination, she must have a license to practice. This means a new series of steps are required, forcing her to pay another set of tolls run by a different group of institutions whose work is supported by yet another set of entrepreneurial actors.

Nurses must prove that they are licensed before they can practice, and their licenses have to be recognized in the state or country where they wish to work. As in the case of physician licensure, there is no internationally recognized and accepted standard that governs nurse licensure. Each nation (or state or province depending on the country's regulations) determines the educational preparation and qualifications required. To complicate matters further, within nursing there are various categories or levels of practice. There are what are called licensed practical nurses in the United States or enrolled nurses in the United Kingdom and Australia—nurses who go to school for a shorter period of time (usually one year), have a reduced scope of practice, and, depending on the assigned responsibilities and employment setting, work under the supervision of the registered nurse. The registered, qualified, or professional nurse (who must study for two to four years before taking a licensure exam) is the most strictly monitored and regulated, using nationally or provincially agreed norms of education and practice.

Before they can practice in another country, its authorized regulatory body has to check the credentials and skills of the registered nurse applicants. Where mutual recognition agreements exist between countries—in other words, the regulatory bodies of the source and host country have formally recognized that their nursing education programs are essentially the same—the applicant nurse will automatically get her license to practice upon request. Between countries where such an agreement has not been reached, careful review of the applicant's transcripts, diplomas, and work references will be undertaken. During the screening process the nurse may have to submit a written application, present herself for a personal interview, take an exam, and/or supply evidence that she has undergone a supervised clinical placement for a specified period of time. In most countries, she must also prove that she can competently communicate in the language of that country.

National licensing exams may have a high failure rate for foreign-educated nurses; 50 percent of foreign graduates have been known to fail the Australia test.[33] Some countries have opted to introduce a pretest. This inserts an additional level of screening in order to identify candidates who are more likely to pass the actual licensing exam. Licensing exams tend to be given in the destination country, while pretests are offered in a variety of sites around the world and are often less expensive. The pretest decreases the cost for the nurse unlikely to pass the actual licensing exam. It also spares the licensing board the problems of dealing with high failure rates—that is, the tasks of developing confidential (high-security) exams and organizing test sites for significant numbers of applicants who have poor chances of passing. While it may be a financial advantage to have as many as possible take the test, since they are charged an exam fee, this is not the primary purpose. In the search for a foreign workforce, it is more cost-effective to guarantee space at the test sites for persons likely to succeed. It also reduces the numbers of persons who fail the exam and thus the level of discontent.

In the United States, the National Council of State Boards of Nursing (NCSBN) is a not-for-profit organization whose membership is comprised of the boards of nursing in the fifty states, the District of Columbia, and five US territories. One of its major responsibilities is the development and administration of the licensing exam for registered nurses (NCLEX-RN examination).[34] Passing the NCLEX exam is a necessary step in obtaining one's license to practice nursing in the United States. It has also, however, become a proxy for academic achievement and clinical expertise. NCLEX holders are often viewed more favorably when applying for entry to post-basic education programs abroad.

Each state is responsible for administering the licensing exam, and the fees charged vary from $20 to $160. Current NCSBN products range from online continuing education courses to review courses to help nurse candidates prepare for their exam. According to their website, NCSBN "produces important resources for boards of nursing, nursing faculty, nursing students, practicing nurses and others involved in the nursing community."[35] While it is a nonprofit organization, this is an income-generating enterprise, and the group markets its services and products to a large number of target populations.

In the 1960s, faced with very high failure rates (80–85 percent) among foreign-educated nurses taking the NCLEX-RN, a pretest was recommended. The introduction of such a test added a new service, which was developed and is managed by an independent group of employees and management, the Commission on Graduates of Foreign Nursing Schools (CGFNS).

CGFNS describes itself as an immigration-neutral nonprofit organization that screens foreign-educated nurses (and several other health professionals) seeking temporary or permanent US occupational visas. Although CGFNS is a not-for-profit organization, it is nonetheless a moneymaking enterprise. The organization's revenues increased from $2.5 million in 1996 to $18 million in 2004, almost all from fees charged to nurses. Historically these fees have been relatively high for foreign nurses. In the late 1970s the fee represented as much as six weeks' salary for certain nurses.[36] As of January 1, 2004, the application fee for the Credentials Verification Service of CGFNS for New York State was increased to $275.[37] CGFNS can charge these fees and generate this kind of income because it has had a virtual monopoly on the exam market. As a prerequisite for taking the licensing exam (NCLEX-RN), forty states have legislation that requires foreign-educated nurses to pass the specific pretest developed by CGFNS. For a foreign nurse, in fact, just scoring well on the CGFNS exam has in itself become a prestigious accomplishment.

Some foreign nurses who have no intention of ever emigrating take the CGFNS exam in order to upgrade their curriculum vitae and employment applications in their own country. This has become a selling point that has helped CGFNS expand its market. According to Ellen Sanders, past CGFNS president, the exam is "a credential even if the nurse does not migrate. When the CGFNS testing center was established in India, it raised the prestige of nursing in the country."[38] Passing the qualifying exam has had unexpected advantages. Barbara Nichols, CGFNS chief executive officer, says their certificate has even been mentioned in personal ads placed by young women searching for suitable marriage partners. The CGFNS certificate has become a proxy indicator for professional status and income-generating potential.

CGFNS activities are not limited however to the screening of foreign-educated health professionals. What began as an organization with a national focus is rapidly becoming a global enterprise. It now provides consultation services to a wide range of other countries. CGFNS created the International Consulting and Educational Service (ICE), which promises to "assist those in need of consultation on international standards, education and licensure/registration for health care professions around the world."[39]

In 2000 the commission acquired its newest division, the International Consultants of Delaware. The ICD is said to be "a credentialing agency evaluating international educational documents and providing their US equivalents. These equivalents are used to assist individuals in obtaining additional education, employment and immigration visas, as well as licensing and certification for healthcare professionals."[40] "Nonprofit" and "in-come-generating" are not contradictory, as CGFNS has proven.

In general, each country has a different credentialing process. The proce-dures may change over time responding to new professional, labor market, trade, and immigration policy. In federated countries, specific states or provinces may impose different standards and credentialing mechanisms. For example, North Dakota requires that the minimum educational prepa-ration for the registered nurse is the bachelor's degree (as opposed to an as-sociate's degree or diploma, which is accepted in all other states). Suffice it to say that the recognition of qualifications in the destination country, state, or province is required if nurses wish to work there as professionals. Failure to do this condemns them to work in nonprofessional occupations or aban-don the health care sector.

Consider the experience of Denise Duvoisin, the US-educated Swiss nurse introduced earlier. At one stage of her life, she traveled to Spain and wished to find employment there as a nurse. Her US bachelor's degree in nursing clearly equipped her to meet the national regulatory requirements. Expecting the process to be a formality, she was surprised when bureau-cratic procedures took much longer than expected. She quickly had to find alternative employment to survive financially. She refused to work as a nursing auxiliary and began to look for other options. Because native speakers were in very high demand and well paid, Duvoisin found a job almost immediately in the private sector giving English language lessons. The health sector missed the opportunity of having a qualified nurse join their ranks.

Not all nurses are as lucky as Denise Duvoisin in finding alternative em-ployment. Many are naïve about the bureaucratic process associated with registration and applying for jobs and work permits. A wide range of for-profit enterprises and nonprofit organizations are involved in the registra-tion process—some ready to support, others geared to exploit. Independent consultants, organizations, and enterprises, for example, are ready and will-ing—for a fee—to help migrating nurses who intend to reregister in a for-eign country. Not all of these businesses will be legitimate and will provide the services promised.

In 2003 CGFNS disseminated an alert when it was notified that individ-uals and training-center employees falsely claimed they had access to the CGFNS qualifying exam. The commission took pains to explain that "CGFNS assures very tight security surrounding the qualifying exam. No individuals or organizations have access to the qualifying exam. Those who claim to have the exam are not being truthful and aim to take advan-tage of the nurse applicant."[41] The alert announced that CGFNS does not operate, license, endorse, or recommend any training, review, online courses, schools, or study materials that claim to prepare applicants for the CGFNS qualifying exam. Clearly, the individuals involved were trying to exploit credulous nurse applicants.

In yet another alert sent out in 2004, CGFNS warned about a company called Visa Assist Program (VAPI) of Largo, Florida, which claimed to have filed all the required forms and documentation with the Department of Homeland Security and was providing certified visa certificates not only for nurses but for other health care professionals as well. The VAPI marketing letter added that as of July 26, 2004, the certified visa certificate was mandatory for all foreign health care providers who wish to enter, work, or remain employed legally in the United States, thus targeting foreign-educated nurses in the United States as well as those abroad.[42]

The CGFNS alert clearly stated that VAPI had, in fact, not been authorized to evaluate credentials or issue certificates under section 343 of the Illegal Immigration Reform and Immigrant Responsibility Act. CGFNS reported this false and misleading claim to the Department of Homeland Security and attempted to inform all health care professionals and all health care organizations about the scam. But was this alert broadcast quickly enough worldwide to prevent countless nurses from being duped and exploited?

In the United Kingdom, there have been similar problems with adaptation programs or supervised clinical placements that are meant to validate migrant nurses' qualifications and help them navigate the barriers to practice once they are in the country. The United Kingdom, being part of the European Union, is bound by the EU nursing directives to automatically recognize nurses' qualifications obtained in any other member state. This expanding and important regulatory framework will be covered in detail in chapter 5.

When a non-EU migrant nurse enters the United Kingdom, she can only practice as a professional nurse once the Nursing and Midwifery Council (NMC) has screened her educational records and certified her qualifications. After this review, the NMC may decide that an adaptation period (supervised clinical placement) of three to twelve months is warranted. The placement is neither a course nor an exam. It is meant to be a period of support and supervision by a named mentor. The NMC, however, will only register nurses whose clinical placements have been evaluated and certified by a higher education institution delivering pre- and postregistration programs. Furthermore, to obtain the stamp of approval, nurses must enter placements where the ratio of nurses to supervisors does not exceed a predetermined maximum. Clinical placements or adaptation programs are not in adequate supply. Independent agencies have discovered a new market—finding clinical placement programs and charging foreign-educated nurses a fee for this service.

If an adaptation period is required, nurses have two years in which to undertake the supervised clinical placement and get a mentor's or supervisor's approval. Until nurses are officially registered, they are paid as nursing auxiliaries in hospitals or nursing homes, either in the public or the private sector (generally on B grade instead of the higher-paying D grade given to new nurse graduates). According to Keith Connell, director of a UK-based agency, "Employers are under no obligation to start their periods of assessment within a specified time, so a nurse can be kept waiting for nine months working as a care assistant."[43]

One nurse explained what it was like to work in a nursing home during this so-called adaptation period. "It was strange when I worked in a nursing home. . . . I was doing carers' jobs [the work of auxiliaries] which was inappropriate. But if there was no cover [charge nurse], I was told I had to stay until cover could be arranged."[44]

This nurse was unofficially and temporarily promoted to a registered nurse (that is, made to take on higher level responsibilities) when it was convenient and then as quickly demoted when her services were no longer critically required. Which raises a question: When is a nonregistered migrant nurse a nurse? Answer: When there is no UK-registered nurse available.

As long as these employees fall short of the registration criteria, their employers have access to nursing staff with professional-level skills at the price of auxiliary staff. A Royal College of Nursing senior employment relations adviser, Verity Lewis, explains that the difference between pre- and postregistration salaries "provides a powerful disincentive for some employers to help their staff successfully complete their adaptation."[45]

The adaptation maze that separates the migrant nurse from permanent employment in a decent job with decent pay actually benefits employers. The whole process builds a perverse incentive into the system when their internationally recruited nurses fail to meet registration requirements. Failure is, unfortunately, not uncommon since some unscrupulous educational and supervision services seem to have an equally perverse incentive—financial gain—to sabotage the process.

Over the past decade, some internationally recruited nurses contracted with facilities that falsely claimed to provide them with legitimate preregistration placements. Imagine the nurses' chagrin and frustration when, their adaptation period finished, they were told that they had to start all over again in an audited facility. What had happened? The NMC revealed that, having been misled by the employer and by the education and training agency, thirty-four nurses paid at least £1,200 for what they thought was a legitimate adaptation program—an official university audited clinical placement. At the end of their training period, the UK regulatory body was obliged to refuse them registration because the training was considered inadequate. While some of the nurses had been placed in audited nursing homes, others had not. To make matters even more complicated, the training company had placed some nurses in approved facilities, but too many nurses per facility. The NMC then decided it had exceeded the number of nurses the home was authorized to supervise and thus deemed their training to be inadequate.[46]

In other isolated cases, supervisors have accepted bribes to facilitate a nurse's admission to the NMC register. Currently, a supervisor is under investigation after having approved the registration of 113 internationally recruited nurses in a period of three months—a physical impossibility if proper supervision is to take place.

Another problem occurred in the United Kingdom when a large group of Chinese nurses were refused registration at the end of their adaptation period. The migrant nurses had been allowed into the country, had been given jobs in health facilities, and had worked for a number of months. The women were, nonetheless, told they had not advanced enough in their English language skills to be registered and practice as professional nurses. These nurses now found themselves trapped in poorly paid and lower-skilled work. Who was to blame for their failure? Was it the employer who may not have supported the learning process? Was it faulty teaching methods of their instructors? When they were approved for employment, were they given overly optimistic estimates of the time it would take to meet their language objectives? Or was it lack of aptitude or concentration on the part of the nurses themselves? Quality assurance is fundamental in health care and applicable in the provision of all services. Protection against misleading advertisement and abusive commerce is needed, especially with vulnerable populations that have difficulty communicating and getting access to the proper authorities. For many migrant nurses, however, it is not there.

Given the number of nurses who enter the preregistration process, professional regulatory organizations like the NMC have insufficient staff to vet each agency, each training program, and each hospital or health facility in which nurses are trained and ostensibly supervised. In fact, the NMC is not given this mandate—the evaluation of clinical placement performance takes place once the nurses claim that their adaptation periods have been successfully completed. There are thus clear pitfalls in the reregistration process with opportunities for exploitation at every step of the way. It is not surprising that a major consultation is taking place to review roles, responsibilities, procedures, and mechanisms.

Canadian provincial governments have recognized these problems and yet have announced their intention to facilitate the entry of skilled workers from other countries. As in most industrialized countries, the number of foreign-educated nurses applying for licensure is increasing. In 2001 Canadian nursing regulatory bodies received over 4,400 applications and 1,689 international applicants wrote the Canadian Registered Nurse Examination (CRNE), a 239 percent increase from 1998. The Canadian Nurses Association (CNA) is working with the federal government to ensure that the recruitment and integration of nurses from other countries respect the licensure requirements for nursing in Canada.

According to the CNA a regulatory framework under the trademark *LeaRN* will guide the process for registration and integration of international applicants. This set of materials includes "a preparation and study guide for the licensing exam, the CRNE Readiness Test™, plus links to Web-based courses on communication skills, language proficiency, nursing practice in Canada and ethics. *LeaRN* resources will also include information on immigrating to Canada, nursing regulation, the Canadian healthcare system and the nursing labor market."[47] Growing reliance on internationally recruited nurses is creating new programs that respond to, and ironically sometimes induce, demand for new services. Existing regulatory bodies either meet these challenges, thus legitimizing their leadership positions in the field, or face competition from entrepreneurs looking for a market niche providing support services to foreign nurses wishing to work abroad.

Step Three: Visas and Work Permits

Once the education maze is negotiated, nurses must obtain the proper visas and work permits to allow them to actually get a job in the country. Their ability to navigate this particular obstacle course is frequently influenced by dynamic and powerful political, social, and economic forces.

Over the past decade, health care downsizing has been one of the global realities that has shaped nurse migration. Consider, the US example. Between 1990 and 1995 the H-1A temporary visa was the major vehicle of entry to the United States for migrant nurses. This visa was introduced in 1990, during a major nursing shortage, to facilitate the migration of foreign-educated nurses. The dramatic downsizing of health facilities, mergers of hospitals, and the introduction of managed care changed the situation in 1995, suddenly creating an oversupply of nurses.[48] Many nurses were given pink slips and faced unemployment. US nurses quickly lobbied to protect their jobs and career opportunities. As the need for new international recruits was greatly reduced, the H-1A visa was withdrawn, once again confirming that domestic policies continue to drive and shape the labor market.

Since 1995, nurses who want to go to the United States are eligible for three types of temporary work visas; the H-1C, TN (Trade NAFTA) status, and the H-1B. The H-1C visas are very limited in number and allow foreign nurses to work in the United States for a maximum of three years and only in designated underserved areas. The TN visa is linked to the North American Free Trade Agreement (NAFTA), which applies only to nurses coming from Mexico and Canada. These visas are issued for one year and are renewable for multiple one-year periods. The H-1B visa is a temporary US visa that applies only to workers with "specialty occupations," usually those that require at least a bachelor's degree.[49] Only one state (North Dakota) requires a university degree for licensure and has the unique privilege of granting H-1B visas for nursing positions. The difficulties in getting any of the three temporary work visas have encouraged nurses who wish to work in the United States to apply for permanent residency (green card) rather than migrate for a limited period of time.

Applications for permanent residence may be submitted in parallel to applications for temporary visas. The pressure on recruiters to find ways for migrant nurses to enter the United States has led them to exploit the H-1B visa option as much as possible. Some believe that recruiters will try to use North Dakota as a pit stop or holding station on the route to work in other states. A temporary H-1B visa will allow university-qualified foreign nurses to work in North Dakota while they wait for their green card applications to be processed in another state. Once their permanent residency papers are in hand, they can fan out and work in any one of the fifty states. North Dakota may benefit from this special status and become a gateway state or a labor-market revolving door created by the new immigration policy.[50]

Changes in visa requirements and the professional screening process may stimulate business activity but may also change the interrelationships and dynamics of the major players. As far as foreign-educated nurses are concerned, CGFNS has traditionally been designated as the official agency for screening. Regulations issued in September 2003 break the virtual monopoly that CGFNS has enjoyed since 1977 as the only organization offering a nursing pretest service in the United States.[51] This may have spin-off effects, either limiting the scope of CGFNS action or the reverse, encouraging diversification and a wider range of services. According to one journalist, financial backers are eager to find a competitor to challenge CGFNS—proof that this is an attractive income-generating area. For the time being, however, there is no sign of serious bids. Introducing competition and audits in the pretest market may have unexpected results for all those concerned—including foreign nurses who may find themselves less out of pocket if exam fees are reduced in order to gain a competitive edge in the expanded market.

As the case of Rachel Turner suggested, the rise of international terrorism has also influenced global migration. After the 2001 attacks on the World Trade Center in New York, the United States dramatically tightened its immigration policy and created the Department of Homeland Security. In September 2003, this department issued a rule that adds even more complexity to the migration process and thus provides greater opportunities for new business initiatives. This rule requires nurses and certain other health care workers from overseas to obtain a certificate from an approved credentialing organization verifying their education, training, licensure, and experience before they enter the United States. The rule will be applied whether the nurses trained in the United States or overseas. Immigration attorneys expect the requirement to delay the immigration and credentialing procedures by three to six months for foreign-born nurses, thus creating an additional commercial niche for immigration lawyers or other intermediaries who promise to facilitate or accelerate the process.[52]

Since January 2005, the National Council of State Boards of Nursing offers the NCLEX-RN licensing exam in Seoul, London, and Hong Kong. While all current state licensure requirements still apply, international administration of the NCLEX-RN will accelerate access of foreign graduates to the US labor market, and it will minimize the overall cost to candidates by eliminating the need to travel to the United States each time they must test.[53] It will also create employment for the administrating enterprise and most likely decrease the revenue, workload, and workforce of CGFNS, if the commission's scope of activity remains the same.

Revised rules and regulations have a direct impact on the assessment of credentials, and international trade agreements also bring about change. Scrutiny of qualifications is a constantly evolving process influenced by the external environment as well as by professional concerns for quality care and patient safety. Registration or professional regulation is under review in many countries, and changes are likely in the coming years.

Recruitment Initiatives

As they try to negotiate the complex barriers to immigration, the majority of nurses generally deal directly with the employer for jobs and work permits. Many nurses have commented that they get a better deal when they avoid intermediaries—it is less costly and there are fewer unpleasant surprises. Most nurses learn about job opportunities through family, friends, colleagues, or advertisements. Migrant nurses may, however, go to the United States without prearranged employment. They can enter the country as a tourist, a student, or a spouse; their first stop is usually a city where they can stay with family members. Then they begin searching for a job.

Nurses often find jobs through word of mouth, a grapevine created by four decades of aggressive recruitment. When direct links with a diaspora do not exist, nurses have recourse to newspapers, nursing journals, and the Internet, where they can read advertisements placed by hospitals or international recruitment agencies. Job advertisements are a conspicuous feature of the migration superhighway. A nurse in India, Mauritius, or Finland picks up the May 2004 edition of the *American Journal of Nursing* and discovers that Beresford Blake Thomas, a staffing agency, is publicizing "exciting positions throughout the USA, Canada, and around the world" and declaring that "city living can be good for your wealth . . . and your career!"

An Indonesian nurse, on the other hand, may go to the *Australian Nursing Journal,* a publication peppered with recruitment ads. The back cover of the February 2004 issue is divided between one ad that tries to lure foreign nurses to Australia while another seeks Australian nurses who want to leave the country. "A career choice that gets your heart racing," the Malvern Nurses agency tells the foreign nurse who wants to move down under, while Worldwide Healthcare informs Australian nurses that now is "a time to fly, a time to play, a time for a change!" The *World of Irish Nursing* carries an ad encouraging nurses to work abroad and reach for their dreams. The *Canadian Nurse* of May 2000 carries an ad recruiting their professionals to Switzerland, "the heart of Europe."

A South African nurse need not bother searching foreign professional journals. In the June 2003 issue of the South African journal *Nursing Update* she will find an ad, again placed by Beresford Blake Thomas, promising "a world of opportunities at your fingertips." Job advertisements, many of them international ads, are a significant source of income for professional nursing journals and their sponsoring organizations. This in spite of the potential conflict of interest between organizations sponsoring these publications and hospitals and recruitment agencies draining precious nurses from their native lands. Many of the organizations that sponsor nursing publications, like the Democratic Nursing Organization of South Africa, the American Nurses Association, and the Royal College of Nursing, have taken official positions supporting the retention of nurses and protesting or expressing concern about foreign recruitment. All nurses' organizations recognize the right of the individual to migrate, and one of the key objectives of journals is to inform. It is very difficult to ban employment advertising without infringing these rights or this mission. Since journals support themselves from advertising revenue, they may also risk bankruptcy, since few other sources of income are as lucrative. Nurse leaders, especially in developing countries in Africa, have had to deal with the dilemma of ads that may further deplete an already reduced workforce. The conflict exists even in industrialized countries, where journals have numerous alternative sources of advertisement revenue. *Kai Tiaki,* the journal of the New Zealand Nurses Organization, regularly publishes a disclaimer adjacent to advertisements for overseas positions. It states that the magazine accepts advertisements for nurse recruitment agencies but cannot guarantee the quality of the service provided by them.[54]

The growth of employment advertising and travel nursing have yielded profitable travel- and leisure-oriented magazines that target this expanding subscriber market. Employment advertising is such a lucrative commercial activity that publishers are launching new journals completely devoted to this purpose. In one UK initiative, the publisher plans to send a free magazine to the homes of the 650,000 health professionals in the Nursing and Midwifery Council's register. The source of revenue for this publication will come exclusively from the health care facilities placing the ads, prices starting at £500 per issue. Interested parties will also have their paid advertisements made available for one month on the publisher's website.

This type of advertisement is not limited to journals but can also be found on the web. TravelNursing.com promises to "make it easy—simply fill out an application and send it to the nation's most reputable travel nursing organizations with a single click of the mouse. It's free, there's no obligation, and it's 100% confidential." Nurses are reassured that this website's travel partners have been in business for the last twenty years. They are then asked if they are ready to start travel nursing, and if they assent, they are led through seven steps: choosing a travel nurse company, completing an application, talking to a recruiter, choosing a destination, conducting a telephone interview with the facility, accepting the assignment, and "away you go!"[55]

Other Spin-off Services

Once the foreign-educated nurse receives her employment contract, license to practice, and work permit, the actual move needs to be organized. Getting the nurse from the source country to the destination country demands transport and perhaps relocation of furniture to the new accommodation. Businesses will be required to assist with bookings, the actual travel, storage or moving, finding and then renting a place to live, and local transport. In some cases recruitment agencies take responsibility for many of these; in others the employer or the migrant nurse must do so.

Chris Spencer, a New Zealand nurse working in Canada, found that a relocation allowance is preferable to having airfare paid. "For those needing to buy a car and rent a house, the initial outgoings amount to thousands of dollars and changing this amount of money is unnecessarily expensive."[56] Regardless of who makes the arrangements, a great deal of money is involved. Employees in a wide range of enterprises outside the health sector provide these services, and their livelihood depends in part on nurse migration.

Some Middle Eastern countries, for example, recruit expatriate health personnel to provide high-quality health services that their own populations cannot deliver. They then house the international staff in separate residential compounds, limiting the contacts between expatriates and the local inhabitants. Staff is fed, lodged and entertained in isolated "villages." "Life was strange in Saudi Arabia," recalls Ann Baird, a British nurse we met earlier. "Almost all the staff lived on site, so it was, in a way, quite incestuous. People said it was very artificial, which it was on one level. However, as we all lived and worked on the same site, you got to know people really well."

Travel agencies also get a boon when more nurses migrate. In the 1960s and 1970s Philippine travel agencies worked with US sponsoring hospitals to target nurses in their advertising. These agencies doubled as Filipino nurses purchased airplane tickets to go abroad. Many travel agencies offered seductive "fly now, pay later" packages, but some nurses found there was a hitch. Once the nurses arrived in the United States, the agencies charged them 12 percent interest rates.[57] Counting on the periodic visits of large groups of migrant workers to major source countries, tour agencies and airlines still organize special vacation packages or charter flights for important public holidays.

To accelerate the process of employing internationally recruited nurses, health facilities have turned to specialized immigration lawyers. As governments try to negotiate between the sometimes conflicting demands of employers and workers, and as they balance their professional regulatory functions and stricter security measures to combat international terrorism, they enact increasingly complex webs of rules, regulations, procedures, and documentation requirements written in highly technical legalese. Navigating this bureaucratic maze is taking more and more time. All of this encourages migrants and employers to seek advice from law firms that specialize in immigration. These law firms help nurses grapple with the differences between tourist versus student visas, temporary versus permanent visas, and special need versus specialty occupations. Requirements and application procedures for each type of visa are carefully negotiated, and the purpose, time frame, and target group are decided by various government departments such as immigration, trade, and health in the case of nurses. Needless to say, only a specialist can easily master this legalese. To do so, skilled immigration lawyers may charge up to three thousand dollars per employee for legal fees and visa processing. Entire law firms have been devoted to immigration matters and established to deal with these complex procedures and increasing demands for skilled international migrants.

Everyday transactions can present business opportunities. For nurses far from home, international phone calls are an important means of maintaining contact with family and friends. Telephone companies offer special promotional packages to international migrants to attract their patronage. In many countries phone companies vie for migrants' business in the fiercely competitive environment that has accompanied the privatization of the telecommunications industry.

Another enormous business opportunity is assisting migrant nurses to send their money back home. In 2004 workers' remittances sent through formal banking channels are estimated to have reached $100 billion, which is why advertisements encouraging international residents to send money home to the family are common sights in migrant-rich areas, including the London subway, which is used daily by thousands of migrant workers.

For migrant nurses, sending money home can be a costly enterprise. Some of the intermediary enterprises now responsible for money transfers such as banks and post offices may charge up to 25 percent commission. Money orders, money transfers, official checks, and gift certificates constitute a growing business as the number of international migrants increases. The cost of a $200 transfer ranges from 13 to 20 percent. To give an idea of how onerous these charges are for migrant nurses and their families in developing countries, the World Bank estimates that a reduction of five percentage points in fees could generate annual savings of $4 billion to $5 billion for all overseas workers. If migrants, including nurses, could send that extra money home, it would increase their families' income and help spur economic growth in their home countries.[58]

The transfer of remittances now represents a significant part of the workload of post office employees in both the sending and receiving countries. Depending on the location of the post office and its clientele, financial transactions may dominate, taking the place of traditional duties directly linked with communication (e.g., letters, packages).

Some governments are encouraging the creation of different types of bank accounts for the transfer of remittances, each one accommodating the specific purpose intended for the money sent. For example, the automatic payment of recurring bills, such as monthly rent or mortgage payments on a house occupied by elderly parents still living in the home country, would require a different type of account than money reserved for future investment or as collateral to open a business. Often the migrant worker earns a salary paid in hard currency (e.g., dollars or pounds) that is relatively stable in value, whereas the currency in the home country (e.g., the South African rand or the Philippine peso) may suffer from severe devaluation through high inflation rates or government-imposed currency exchange rates. It is often in the migrants' interest to keep money saved in the hard currency. Banks from the industrialized and the developing countries are now creating partnerships in order for accounts in the home country to be maintained in hard currency, thus eliminating the risk of loss in purchasing power. Satisfying the clients' needs will promote business by encouraging the formal transfer of funds, an advantage for banks in both the source and the destination country charging fees for the service.

Competition has already started to reduce fees for money transfers. Western Union now charges $10 for a $200 transfer from the United States to Mexico and $22 for sending the same amount to the Philippines. While they represent a reduction, Dilip Ratha, an economist for the World Bank, believes these fees are still too high, as the true cost is a flat rate of $2–$3.[59] Lower charges may encourage workers to make greater use of the formal transfer channels. This would give banks and private money courier companies access to the untapped pool of $180 billion and more estimated to move informally from country to country. The attraction, even at a reduced profit margin, is clear.

Following a negotiation with the Mexican government and as part of a marketing campaign targeting Latin American workers in the United States, a group of banks agreed to lower the transfer commission rate to 5 percent. As a result a further $1–$2 million per year reaches relatives and investment projects in Latin America.[60] Similarly, three banks in Paris offer a special transfer scheme to Côte d'Ivoire, Mali, and Senegal; in 1999 they officially transferred $24 million to Senegal alone.[61] Remittances are changing the work and life patterns of thousands—senders, receivers, and intermediaries.

Recruitment Agencies

None of these commercial opportunities would be possible without the major business player in international nurse migration—nurse recruitment agencies. Recruitment agencies are for-profit organizations that link the employer who wishes to hire staff and the nurse who is looking for a job. Some hospitals and other health facilities have their own headhunters, of course. Others depend on recruitment agencies that either have staff established in the various source countries or subcontract to local recruitment agencies.

The hospital or health care institution usually pays the agency a fee for each nurse hired. Out of that money, the agency pays its overhead and the travel and application expenses of each nurse it recruits, including travel expenses, exam fees, tutoring, and housing expenses in the destination country. Some agencies advance money to cover these expenses and include them in the bill given to an employer. Some expect the nurse to reimburse the agency once she has begun to work.

There are hundreds, perhaps even thousands, of recruitment agencies across the globe. A trip to the web or a cursory glance at nursing journals reveals a baffling array. While many agencies are legitimate and responsibly run, they have a vested interest in making as much money as the market will bear from every contract they sign. Since no designated body or organization regulates or monitors the recruitment process, the traditional market motto—buyer beware—applies. Each individual nurse has to be mindful of the conditions set by the contracts. These contracts are legal documents, which, once signed, may put the nurse under burdensome obligations. As more and more nurses embark on their excursions using the migration superhighway, the cases of exploitation have multiplied. Contracts are manipulated, human liberties threatened, and blatant fraud is not uncommon.

The often urgent need of employment, especially employment abroad with the promise of higher salaries, makes migrant nurses particularly eager to accept contract conditions without necessarily taking the time to fully investigate the implications or consequences. According to Seny Lipat, past president of the Philippine Nurses Association of America, many cases of exploitation could be avoided if nurses would read the fine print on their contracts and consider the implications carefully.[62] The reality, however, is that "the evolving migration infrastructure of agents and brokers that moves workers over borders takes a significant share of the earnings gap that motivates people to migrate, often 20 to 30% of migrant earnings, which often leaves migrants with lower wages and worse conditions than other workers where they are employed."[63]

Whatever the reason, many migrant nurses are employed under false pretenses or misled as to the conditions of work and possible remuneration and benefits. In the case of international career moves, the difficulty of verifying the terms of employment is increased when distance, language barriers, and cost are added. While exploitation may already begin in the source country, it can occur at any number of points along the recruitment process.

In the late 1990s a thirty-three-month investigation dubbed Operation

Windmill, conducted by the South Plains Texas Visa Fraud Task Force, resulted in the breakup of a major smuggling ring that used fraud and deceit to obtain legitimate temporary H-1A visas—which, we recall, had been withdrawn during the nursing "surplus" of the mid-1990s. The owner of a chain of private nursing homes brought more than five hundred foreign nurses into the United States illegally. These nurses were employed by hospitals, nursing homes, and clinics in thirty-five states across the country, earning substandard wages and living in crowded and at times unsanitary conditions. Some of the registered nurses were hired as nurses' aides and paid hourly rates as low as five dollars per hour.[64] At least fifty of these nurses and their illegal visas were "passed on"—sold—to other unscrupulous recruiters at the price of $1,000 to $1,500 each. At the same time, nurses were charged $7,000 for the privilege of participating in the scheme. This example illustrates the desperation of foreign-educated nurses to work in the United States and the unethical profiteering and exploitation that can occur when legal avenues for migration are restricted.[65]

This fraud also ended up abusing US nurses as well as foreign nurses. According to the Texas Nurses Association, when foreign nurses entered the market and accepted lower wages, the prevailing rate for Texas nurses dropped from $14 per hour to $11 per hour. Coming at a time of massive downsizing in health facilities, the unemployment rate of Texas nurses further increased. Hospitals and other health care facilities, not surprisingly, preferred to employ qualified applicants who accepted the lowest salaries. The estimated loss of salary opportunities for US nurses was calculated to be more than $13 million.[66] Although it stretches the imagination to conceive of health care facilities as trafficking in human beings, it seems that "passing on" skilled professionals may be as profitable as drug smuggling.[67]

Filipino nurses, who have the longest history with migration, may also have the longest history of abuse. In the Philippines, many recruitment agencies charge the nurses a fee, even though this practice is illegal under Philippine law. In one case, four Filipino nurses had to pay $750 each for two interviews in Manila (the equivalent of four months' wages) with no guarantee of getting a job in a Scottish hospital.[68] Lack of government enforcement of the law, combined with government encouragement of migration and high national unemployment, obliged nurses to pay the fee. What is even more disturbing is the fact that agencies that charge nurses such fees may, in fact, be double billing. On top of the money they receive in fees from nurses, they may collect more money from hospitals or health systems who hire the nurses they recruit.

Other forms of duplicity may occur. Nurses may have discussed payment of travel expenses to the destination country and thought they had reached an agreement that the recruitment agency would pay their expenses. When the nurses arrive in the destination country, they find that the cost is either deducted from their paychecks or invoiced by the recruitment agency. Sometimes agencies will add on interest rates if the full amount cannot be paid immediately.[69]

Some agencies try to smuggle nurses into the United States by bringing them in illegally through Mexico. If caught, they go to jail and, in most cases, are deported. In the Philippines, bogus, fly-by-night agencies have charged nurses for services that they will never provide. When the nurses come for a progress report, the agency no longer exists and their money is gone. Less publicized but similar scams have been reported in other countries. Indian nurses were "duped by a fictitious recruitment agency promising jobs in the UK but which only took the recruitment fees. Some Ghanaian nurses signed up to register with one recruitment agency only to later discover that the agency representative had stolen their money."[70]

Another vehicle for abuse is the accommodation charge. A recent scandal broke out in Scotland where the owner of a recruitment agency was charging exorbitant rent for flats sublet to his agency. In one case, four nurses were crammed into a two-bedroom apartment, each charged an exorbitant price. While the average rent for a similar apartment was £395, the nurses together ended up paying £1,100 per month, three times the going rate. In addition, the agency offered the nurses a loan to help pay for the advance rent and deposit as well as a relocation fee. Once the rent, council tax, loan repayment, revenue tax, and national insurance were deducted from their salaries, these nurses were left with £8 per day for daily expenses, including transport and food. A UNISON (UK public-sector trade union) representative called the arrangement "slave labor within the National Health Service."[71]

Exploitation and Abuse

Since 2001, the British public media and professional press have been filled with horror stories of recruitment abuses where foreign nurses have been the victims of what has been labeled a "multi-million-peso, -pound or -dollar industry."[72] According to Allen Reilly (of the UK-based Filipino Community), Filipino nurses have been rescued from "contracts made in hell" and from abusive employers who treat these nurses "more like slaves—all for the sake of profit."[73] The media (including the BBC) have repeatedly reported stories of inferior accommodation at exorbitant rents— for example, five nurses living in a single room above a nursing home, or nurses living in trailers with no toilet facilities. In one case, the nurses were expected to use the toilets of a nearby pub, except in the morning when it was closed.

Accommodation abuses have also been reported in the United States. To give but one example, eight migrant nurses were allocated a four-bed room in a hospital dormitory. The nurses were then rostered or scheduled to work different shifts so that the beds were in constant use.

Nurses are also given incorrect information about where they may work, the nature of working conditions, and what salary they may receive. Internationally recruited nurses are conscious of—and often nervous about—the fact that working conditions as well as cultural practices may differ from one country to another. Before they sign contracts, their employers or recruiters often promise that they will receive orientation courses to ease them into employment. When the nurses arrive in the destination country, the promised orientation course may never materialize.

One nurse from Australia, who had been promised a decent orientation, started work four days after she arrived in the United Kingdom. In the morning of that first day of employment, she received her uniforms and was expected to be on the ward at one o'clock in the afternoon. Assigned a patient load, she was told to "get on with it." That was it. When orientation is available, they may find that their "teachers" are nursing assistants who cannot give a proper introduction to nurses' work and responsibilities.[74]

Perhaps administrators operate under the common prejudice that a nurse is a nurse is a nurse: Anyone who provides whatever sort of nursing care—whether as a registered nurse, technical nurse, or nursing assistant—is qualified to assign patient workloads and teach nursing skills at the professional level. We will see that this myth has been dispelled by research and that its continued application in practice is dangerous. Or perhaps the prevailing assumption is that a nurse dropped into any health care situation, team structure, and work environment can perform at a quality level from day one. Not providing the promised and required orientation amounts to an exploitation of nurses, and expecting them to provide high-level care without a basic knowledge of the environment, equipment, and procedures is unfair. It increases the vulnerability of both the nurses and the patients under their care during these critical first weeks of work.

The lack of regard for past expertise negates nurses' sense of professional worth and undermines their confidence,[75] making them even more vulnerable to exploitation and discrimination. Nurses who have emigrated to industrialized countries may have run a hospital at home but are told the only way they can stay in the country is by doing domestic work—putting out rubbish, ironing bed linen, or mopping floors in a nursing home.[76] In one case a nursing home owner ordered a nurse to wash his car.[77] Some migrant nurses expecting standard working conditions and nursing responsibilities have complained of abusive treatment and long working hours (fifty to sixty hours per week).

A frequently reported form of exploitation is contract substitution. For example, nurses sign a contract in the Philippines, which then gets approval from the Philippines Overseas Employment Administration. Once on UK soil, they become victims of scare tactics and are forced to sign new contracts that offer less pay and often designate a different place of employment. They may find that the new contract obliges them to work for the facility far longer than expected and that it includes bonding clauses that impose high penalties if they resign before the termination date.

To make sure nurses do not complain to the authorities or report their grievances to trade unions or professional associations, employers have used a variety of intimidation tactics, including the retention of identification and travel documents. Beverly Malone, general secretary of the Royal College of Nursing, explained that "over the last few years the RCN has represented hundreds of internationally recruited nurses who have faced exploitation and discrimination—but we know this is just the tip of the iceberg. Many more are too afraid to take action against their recruiters or employers. We know of cases where nurses have their passports taken away and are threatened with deportation if they complain or try to leave. This is no way to treat human beings."[78]

The substantial interest in international nurse recruitment has encouraged the establishment of a growing number of agencies all looking for a piece of the action. As the numbers go up, the amount of business (or profit margin) for each agency tends to go down. The rising competition between agencies may have a good influence on future recruitment practices. As international recruitment continues, the agencies that maintain a good track record (as evidenced by the fact that nurses they have recruited stay employed for an optimal period of time) will be rewarded with more business. Agencies that break promises, provide inadequate support to the recruited nurse, or perpetrate fraudulent or exploitative practices will earn a poor reputation and be put out of business. Such selection occurs slowly, however. In the meantime new generations of nurses continue to suffer, which is unacceptable.

Competition will never completely solve the urgent problems that global migration creates. Some standardization of good practice, government regulation, and sanctions against misconduct are essential. Moreover, nurses will need help from nursing organizations and unions if they are to navigate the maze of restrictions, requirements, commercial enterprises, and employment hazards that characterize international nurse migration.

Migrant nurses often feel defenseless when they face exploitation. Potential allies are the professional organizations and labor unions whose members are, sometimes, protected by national and international law. Two core instruments of the International Labour Organization are Convention 87, which guarantees workers freedom of association (adopted in 1948), and Convention 98, which, at least in theory, guarantees workers the right to organize and bargain collectively (adopted in 1949). In principle, all workers and all employers have the universally accepted right to freely form and join groups for the promotion and defense of their occupational interests. The reality is different, however, even in societies that claim to be the most democratic. Human Rights Watch monitors freedom of association in the United States. It has recently reported a number of cases in which nursing personnel were intimidated and dismissed because of their efforts to organize the Haitian workforce. In one case Haitian workers were harassed, discriminated against, and finally dismissed for conversing in Creole, which was viewed as a subterfuge to defeat an organizing drive. The rule barring workers from speaking Creole was considered to be a vehicle to limit employees' ability to engage in union activity. The administrative law judge ordered the workers reinstated, as the grounds for dismissal were considered illegal.[79]

Throughout the world, millions of nurses are members of professional associations, nurses' unions, or multidisciplinary trade unions. The primary objectives of all three types of organizations as they relate to nurses are to represent the membership, promote the interests of nurses, and advance the profession. Some nurses have argued that there is a neat distinction between the functions of professional and labor organizations. Professional organizations, they contend, are meant to deal solely with "professional issues" such as nursing education, nursing credentialing, and the delivery of nursing services. Unions, on the other hand, are said to deal only with helping to improve workers' wages and working conditions. Some nurses, particularly in the United States, where the rate of unionization of workers is one of the lowest in the world—8 percent of the private sector and 12 percent in the overall workforce (and 17 percent of the nursing workforce)—believe that nurses, because they are professionals and not blue-collar workers, have no place in a labor union.

Even in the United States, however, there is growing recognition that nurses' concerns are influenced by both professional and labor factors and that for every "professional" issue, there are socioeconomic issues that need to be considered. Similarly, all nurses' labor concerns will be influenced by professional factors. This helps explain why, of those organizations in membership with the International Council of Nurses (comprising national nurses' organizations from 126 different countries), professional unions tend to have the most representative and strongest voluntary membership, developing programs that address both the professional and labor concerns of its members.[80]

The role of professional associations and unions is crucial in safeguarding acquired rights and promoting improvements in pay and working conditions for nurses, including migrants. As we will discuss later at greater length, some unions and professional organizations have taken strong stands to protect migrant nurses. The Royal College of Nursing in the United Kingdom has tried to implement protections for migrant nurses and develop codes of conduct for international employers. Again in the United Kingdom, UNISON has developed a series of measures to protect vulnerable migrant nurses. Some governments and unions have even established a hot line where nurses experiencing exploitation or difficulties may call for ready advice. Because of the strength of Philippine migration, Filipino nurses have established effective organizations like the Philippine Nurses Association of America, which has twenty-eight chapters in the United States. Internationally, they have created the Association of Filipino Nurses in the United Kingdom and the Filipino Nurses Association in Saudi Arabia, among others. In some countries generic migrant associations have been established—for example, the association Filipinos in Rome, which includes Filipino migrants from all walks of life. These associations provide help and support once the migrant nurse arrives in her new country of employment. In the United States we also find organizations such as the National Association of Hispanic Nurses and the Asian American/Pacific Islanders Nurses Association.

Although labor unions can be helpful allies for migrant workers, they are sometimes hampered by prejudice and fear as well as by employers' use of migrant workers in ways that seem designed to alienate veteran employees. Longtime union members, some of whom may have been migrants themselves earlier in their careers, may feel that newly recruited migrant nurses are stealing their jobs, lowering their wages, or unfairly receiving perks and privileges not available to them.

Trade unions have traditionally been wary of migrant workers and of what their presence implies. Internationally recruited nurses have often been perceived as a threat to workers' acquired rights in industrialized countries. One very real fear is that migrants will lower the wages and erode working conditions that nurses have struggled to obtain. While this may not be the case for certain highly paid workers in scarce supply, low-paid unskilled workers in an employer's market tend to suffer. According to Jonathan Power, the impact of the migrant workforce needs to be seriously considered. He argues that "in California, American-born workers have left the state as fast as immigrants have moved in, so extreme has been the impact of immigrants in keeping wages down."[81] The consequences of migration flows need to be monitored and regulated while the rights of workers are defended.

There is no consensus on whether the entry of foreign health professionals will actually depress the wages in the destination country. Increased labor supply tends to do exactly that, but the aggressive competition between countries for health professionals may offset and perhaps create the opposite tendency. A downward pressure on nurses' earnings has the potential for decreasing health costs, however—a definite benefit for the consumer or the public purse. Studies undertaken in a market-driven health system estimate that the gain to consumers (as a percentage of total expenditures on physician services) from physician immigration to the United States ranged from close to 1 percent in 1966 to over 12 percent in 1971.[82] Decreases in the cost of services are of considerable interest to businesses looking for a competitive edge in an increasingly difficult market with decreasing profit margins.

Nursing organizations argue that hiring foreign nurses siphons off money that could be used to increase the pay and improve the working conditions of homegrown veteran staff and to attract more local applicants to the profession. The International Council of Nurses goes even further and condemns the practice of recruiting nurses to countries where authorities have failed to "seriously address problems which cause nurses to leave the profession and discourage them from returning to nursing."[83]

The fact that entrepreneurs have launched so many profitable business ventures is clear evidence that there is money to be made off the migrant nurse. But their profits depend, in part, on the willingness of employers—hospitals and other health care institutions—to advertise in the pages of nursing journals and newspapers, pay agency fees for nurse recruitment, and employ a variety of lawyers, recruiters, and consultants to attract foreign nurses. Studies estimate that it costs between two and three times the nurses' salary to replace a single nurse. According to one US study, replacing a medical surgical nurse, who earns on average $46,800, can cost up to $92,400. Replacing an oncology nurse can cost as much as $145,000.[84] The cost of advertising and recruiting in general is so high that many nurses and their representative organizations have questioned why this money continues to be more consistently invested in recruitment as opposed to retention strategies.

Because they fail to understand the kinds of pressures that some employers or recruitment agencies exert over threatened new immigrant workers who fear they will lose jobs or even be deported, many locally educated nurses may also accuse migrant nurses of passively accepting exploitative working conditions. In fact, the socialization and past experience of many migrant nurses, coupled with the vulnerability they experience in a new country lacking strong support networks, may tend to encourage passive behavior, at least in the beginning. Jane Mendoza*, a migrant nurse from the Philippines and now dean of a prestigious college of nursing in the United States, explains that Asians in general are not assertive—such behavior is not culturally acceptable. A US union militant adds that migrant nurses are often perceived as stuck in culture shock and very alienated. "There are sometimes enormous language barriers, and communication is difficult," she says. "Migrant nurses are more trusting of the hospital and more loyal to the institution. Internationally recruited nurses don't wish to rock the boat. Hospitals assume that they can control a foreign workforce more easily, that foreign recruits will be less involved in job action, more reticent to strike and complain. Employers depress wages in non-unionized facilities with threats that if there are complaints the workers will be replaced."

Having come from precarious and very poor conditions, some migrant nurses may find the substandard pay and working conditions offered in the destination country a whole lot better than what was offered in their homeland. When they recognize that they are being exploited, migrant nurses are understandably fearful of complaining, since they are on temporary visas and dependent on recruitment agencies or employers. Challenging their employer and facing the possibility of deportation or unemployment may not be an acceptable option. Not surprisingly, then, other nurses may fear that the migrants' passivity will encourage employers to renege on or withdraw rights nurses have long struggled to obtain. This often creates tensions between unions and migrant nurses.

While all of this is a source of conflict, attitudes are changing—among all nurses and not just migrants. The first two years in a new country are the most difficult for migrant nurses. When personal and professional lives are secure, migrant nurses tend to become more involved in social and work-related networks, including workers' organizations which, they understand, provide opportunities for personal leadership development.

In his report commissioned by the International Labour Office, Stephen Bach clearly states that "the trade union movement in the majority of countries has shifted its focus away from a protectionist and exclusionary stance in which the dominant concern has been that migrants would erode wages and conditions towards a more open and inclusive perspective towards labor migration." He argues that "this altered stance reflects a belief that immigration is an inevitable component of a more globalized economy and that instead of forcing migrants underground into precarious working

conditions, trade unions should encourage the regulation and normaliza-
tion of migrant working conditions, thereby drawing migrants into union
membership."[85]

Anna Biondi of the International Confederation of Free Trade Unions
agrees that paying greater attention to the plight of migrants is a win-win
situation for unionized nurses in industrialized countries and for the migrant nurses entering the workforce. She goes on to recognize the vital role
migrant workers have played and continue to play in revitalizing the labor
movement worldwide.

The primary source of revenue for unions is the membership fee. The
larger the membership base, the more financially viable will be the organization. Good representation and successful negotiation are critical to retain
workers in membership, but workers must first be approached and convinced to become members. Some workers' organizations are beginning to
include overseas workers in their recruitment campaigns, and some have
even offered migrant nurses low membership fees in order to entice them
into membership.[86]

The New York State Nurses Association negotiated to have migrant
nurses' pay upgraded by taking into account their previous work experience
in the source country. The Malta Union of Midwives and Nurses recently in-
tervened and negotiated equal maternity leave rights for migrant nurses
working on short-term (one-year) contracts. These examples highlight the
unions' change in attitude toward migrant workers. They have become advocates of migrant-specific causes.

The current philosophy of workers' organizations today is to lobby for
the regulation of migration and reach out to migrant workers once they are
in the destination country. But it will take more than unions and professional
organizations to defend the rights of migrant and homegrown nurses while
keeping in mind the safety of the patients both groups serve. Government
action and regulation is also necessary.

There has been some positive action on this front. The International Convention on the Protection of the Rights of All Migrant Workers and Members of Their Families came into being in July 2003.[87] The convention was
adopted by a majority of UN member states in the General Assembly back
in 1990 and needed twenty signatories in order to come into effect. This took
all of thirteen years to happen. Finally enough countries have signed on to
these binding international standards that address the treatment, welfare,
and human rights of migrants as well as the obligations and responsibilities
on the part of source and destination countries. Overall, the convention
seeks to prevent and eliminate the exploitation of migrant workers and
members of their families throughout the entire migration process.

There is not much optimism about the impact of this latest legal instrument, however. It is not considered a "magic formula" because the largest labor-receiving countries have not ratified the convention and cannot be forced to do so. What also undermines its effectiveness is the "reluctance of countries supplying the labor—and hence the most victimized—to agree even among themselves on common standards of labor rights and protection they would want upheld by the receiving countries."[88] The competition between source countries to get their workers employed abroad is tremendous due to the promise of future foreign exchange sent back home.

The twenty-one signatories of the UN convention are Azerbaijan, Belize, Bolivia, Bosnia and Herzegovina, Cape Verde, Colombia, Ecuador, Egypt, El Salvador, Ghana, Guatemala, Guinea, Mexico, Morocco, Philippines, Senegal, Seychelles, Sri Lanka, Tajikistan, Uganda, and Uruguay—all developing countries with the most to gain. The major destination countries, where the majority of the exploitation and recruitment abuses take place, are not signing up, although they were involved in the text development and adoption process. Ratifications of the ILO Convention concerning Migration for Employment (No. 97) and the Convention concerning Migrations in Abusive Conditions and the Promotion of Equality of Opportunity and Treatment of Migrant Workers (No. 143) show similar patterns with developing countries making up more than three-quarters of the signatories.

As we have seen, migrant populations are more vulnerable to exploitation and discrimination. What turns risk into reality is the fact that effective protection and regulation often founder when governments and international bodies fail to effectively balance conflicting vested interests. When this happens, double standards replace harmonization, and nurses may be caught in another maze of competing imperatives and confusing but often ill-considered remedial action. Business is business. When there are financial investments and profits to be made, there is always the risk of abuse. The health sector is not immune to this threat.

Strong economic and professional push factors in the developing countries will continue to generate a pool of nurses ready to migrate. The vested interests, hidden agendas, and double standards of governments, enterprises, agencies, and organizations need to be identified so that migrant nurses can make informed decisions and avoid exploitation

4. Vested Interests, Inconsistencies, Double Standards

When she was thirty-five years old, Ethel Nkosi[†] decided to emigrate from South Africa to the United Kingdom. She had worked in a Johannesburg hospital for ten years. Coming home exhausted after each night shift, Nkosi found she could no longer face the prospect of returning to work the next day. Caring for eighty to ninety patients, trying to address their staggering, unremitting needs, had become more than she could bear. Nkosi was providing the best care possible but constantly was confronted with competing priorities and minimal resources. There was no support staff, and although the country was in the midst of an AIDS epidemic, Nkosi had difficulty even finding protective gloves to guard against blood-borne infections.

One day, violence penetrated the hospital walls. A gang leader was admitted to her ward. Several hours later, a member of another, opposing gang arrived and started shooting at him. Nkosi tried to protect herself and her patients. After it was over, she tried to comfort her patients as best she could. But who was there to comfort and reassure her? Although she was experiencing posttraumatic stress, she had no access to counseling. The threat of violence was always on her mind. A single mother of two young daughters, she was also taking care of a niece, one of the fifteen million HIV/AIDS orphans. Her family depended on her to cope.

Nkosi wanted to get out. A recruitment agency tried to come into her hospital, but the management unceremoniously ejected them because they did not want to lose nurses. So Nkosi went to the Internet and found a job in the United Kingdom. Just as she was preparing to emigrate, however, she heard news that Nelson Mandela had encouraged the United Kingdom to ban the recruitment of South African nurses. This request was seriously being considered. How could this be? she wondered. Why would she be denied the ability to exercise her right to emigrate?

The way individuals like Ethel Nkosi collide with political imperatives is one of the things that make international migration such a complex, multifaceted social phenomenon. The magnitude and direction of migration are constantly changing, often unpredictably, under the influence of legislation, trade, conflicts, and other socioeconomic factors or events in the local and national environments. Even the major players in this dynamic process may differ over time depending on the financial and labor markets.

Policy making, whether at the government or business level, most often occurs within an environment of competing priorities and limited resources. Governments need to protect their migrating workers from the kind of exploitation we saw in the previous chapter. They must also protect the integrity of health care systems and meet the needs of patients. It is often difficult for governments to fulfill both mandates, being pulled and prodded by so many conflicting vested interests. If they help individual nurses like Ethel Nkosi to migrate, patients and the broader health care system may be hurt. If they help the businesses or public sector that depend on nurses, they may fail to protect the nurses themselves. Governments are also influenced by other powerful actors, for example, international financial institutions like the World Bank or International Monetary Fund. Meeting the needs of physicians and physician organizations may conflict with their need to protect often less vocal actors like nurses. Finally, governments are swayed by their need to protect trade balances and to cut or expand federal, state, or provincial budgets. Deciding how to proceed is made all the more difficult because most governments and organizations lack the data upon which sound decision making depends.

Perfect solutions are rare and choices must always be made. Consideration of the short, medium, and long term may lead policy makers to develop different or even conflicting strategies. Nor can health issues be adequately addressed in isolation. For example, the management of road traffic, access to health insurance, food safety, housing, the availability of clean water and electricity, and education all directly affect people's health. But they are usually the responsibility of various departments or organizations that may not coordinate their policies or efforts. Despite their consultations, they may take opposing actions or change the environment so much that a strategy taken by a given institutional actor is rendered inappropriate or ineffective. What is more problematic is that policies frequently focus on the short term because of time pressure, immediate needs, and limited resources. They thus often address the most urgent symptoms rather than the cause of the problem.

In Ghana, for example, the Ministry of Health decided to reintroduce a Senior Registered Nurses program in addition to the three-year diploma courses being offered. The program would provide post-basic specialization courses to enhance the nursing skills so desperately needed by the population. Not only would the graduates of the basic and post-basic programs help fill the ranks of the depleted nursing workforce, but they would provide needed skills to educate the population and care for the significant numbers of HIV/AIDS patients in the country. The Nurses Training College in Bolgatanga was not able to admit new students in October 2001, however, because the Ministry of Finance would not give clearance for the contractor to finish work on a dormitory that was about 80 percent complete.[1]

The interdependence of—and ineffective coordination between—different ministries can make a much-needed project vulnerable and even derail it. The resulting frustration is easy to imagine. If projects are difficult to coordinate at the local, regional, or state level, the complexity at the international level—where multiple countries, cultures, business environments, and government bureaucracies are involved—is almost beyond belief.

So we have an urgent need, fueled by a long-term problem, and too many short-term solutions. Hospitals and health care facilities in most countries around the world are desperate to find nurses. In some countries, it is not unusual to find 20–50 percent of the nurse positions vacant. Patient waiting lists in the public sector are increasing. Health issues have become major campaign items in presidential and legislative elections globally. The issue of patient safety is a growing concern and attracting more and more attention. Members of the public are increasingly holding their elected representatives—from state or provincial legislators to presidents or prime ministers—accountable for the quality of health care services. Even in totalitarian states the citizens' right to health is often at the top of the political agenda.

Although people hesitate to become nurses for many reasons, the stories of the nurses we met in chapter 2 highlight some of the major ones—poor pay and working conditions, inadequate respect from administrators, doctors, and even nursing colleagues, lack of avenues for advancement, and greater opportunities for women in other fields. These are all significant systemic problems that require time, money, and goodwill to address. Few governments or policy makers seem to focus on the root factors that cause and sustain this current shortage. When it comes to public concern about critical nursing shortages, international recruitment is one way that governments or health care bureaucrats—whether in the private or public sector—can, however, appear to be addressing the crisis. In a kind of employment chain reaction, the pool of international recruits to one country is usually taken from another country that is less wealthy. So the United States goes to Ireland, Ireland goes to South Africa, and South Africa, accusing the United

Kingdom of poaching its nurses, reaches out to its neighbors. Health care administrators come to resemble little boys sticking their fingers in multiple dikes to try to stop the flood of water. The absence of a comprehensive and global approach means that, in the inevitable power struggles that arise around this crucial workforce issue, strong vested interests often dominate policy making. This in turn means that double standards become the norm and poor countries and marginal groups often pay penalties that richer ones avoid.

Recruitment Bans

There is no better example of this dynamic than the debate about migration in South Africa. South Africa seems to have one policy when it comes to the international recruitment of its physicians and another for its nurses, both of which play out against the backdrop of an increasingly popular approach to the dilemmas of nurse migration—the recruitment ban.

South Africa is described as a middle-income developing country with an abundant supply of resources and well-developed financial, legal, communications, energy, and transport sectors. Its stock exchange ranks among the ten largest in the world, and its modern infrastructure supports a distribution of goods to all major urban centers in the region.[2] The country, with a population of more than forty-three million, faces the challenge of establishing a public health system that is equitable and accessible to all. Because the new South Africa inherited formidable economic problems from the apartheid era, namely, widespread poverty of disadvantaged groups and a 30 percent unemployment rate, this promise has been very hard to fulfill.

During the apartheid era, hospitals were assigned to particular racial groups and most were concentrated in white areas. There was no real attempt to deliver primary health care to the majority of the population, and the health sector was largely hospital based. Since South Africa's first democratic elections in 1994, the country's discriminatory health system is being transformed. The government has built new community care clinics, upgraded already existing clinics, and introduced mobile clinics in rural areas. Free health care for children under six, and for pregnant or breast-feeding mothers, is now available.[3]

All these improvements have led to a major emphasis on community and home health care. The demand for health professionals to deliver this care nationwide increased practically overnight. The health system, especially in rural areas, had a long history of chronic short-staffing and was highly dependent on foreign-recruited medical personnel. With this new focus on freely accessible primary health care, the workload of employed staff escalated and the need for additional workers became even greater. Nationals however often avoid assignments in rural areas, perceived as hardship posts because of their isolation, chronic understaffing, poor equipment, reduced career opportunities, and difficult working conditions. The public health sector had to turn elsewhere for a solution and actively recruited from the pool of interested health professionals in other countries.

The Commonwealth of Nations is a voluntary association of fifty-four independent sovereign states, each nominally responsible for its own policies, that consult and cooperate in their common interests and in the promotion of world peace. With a total population of 1.7 billion people, the Commonwealth represents almost one-third of the world's population. The Commonwealth also constitutes one of the largest language blocks in the world. A shared common language, colonial past, and history of migration favor the movement of health professionals among the member countries. The United Kingdom, Canada, Australia, and New Zealand, along with the richer developing countries within a given region, are common destinations for all categories of Commonwealth African health professionals.[4] At times, more developed countries within a region act as intermediate destinations for those who may eventually migrate further.

Some southern African countries attract intraregional migrants because of the relatively higher salaries offered to workers of all types, including professional health workers. For example, in 1999 the average monthly pay in US dollar equivalents for junior doctors was $1,161 in Namibia and $1,242 in South Africa, compared to $199 in Ghana and $200 in Zambia.[5] Although salary is not the only factor determining the migration of health professionals, it is a significant influence for people willing to consider an international career move.

Of the total medical workforce in South Africa, 22 percent is expatriate. Compared to neighboring countries like Lesotho and Namibia, the percentage may be smaller (69 percent in Lesotho and 55 percent in Namibia), but the absolute number is significantly higher (6,705 as opposed to 92 and 152).[6] When looking at rural areas exclusively, the percentage increases dramatically. Foreign migrants constitute 78 percent of the rural physicians in South Africa, many of them Africans.[7] The effective functioning of these health systems relies on the ongoing participation of expatriate physicians. Clearly, significant numbers of these physicians come from other African Commonwealth countries that are confronted with an already depleted workforce.

In response to the outcry from many of those countries, South Africa introduced a moratorium on the registration of foreign physicians in 1996. But as demand surged, the moratorium was quickly removed and foreign re-

cruitment reinstated. In contradiction, the government paradoxically refused to grant permanent work permits to physicians from developing
countries.[8] At present the government has again changed its position and is
facilitating the registration of foreign-educated physicians and a government-to-government agreement between South Africa and Cuba has encouraged a massive flow of Cuban physicians to the rural areas of South
Africa.[9]

These additions to the medical workforce have in general been welcomed. There are, however, residual resentments. The foreign, non-Cuban
physicians have expressed some discontent. They say they feel slighted because the government offers Cuban recruits different and somewhat better
conditions. Although their pay is less than South African peers, the Cuban
physicians receive free airfare, lavish welcome banquets, several weeks of
training, and free housing and transportation. In addition, they enjoy a level
of job security not granted to other foreign physicians. For example, Safdar
Malick, a Pakistani physician who is head of anesthesiology at a three-hun-
dred-bed hospital about seventy-five miles from Johannesburg, says, "On
24-hours notice, we can be told, 'We don't need you. You must go.'"[10] Foreign doctors who were working in the rural areas of South Africa long before the Cubans arrived are now leaving en masse.

What was introduced as an ethical solution to the physician shortage in
South Africa may have medium- or long-term negative consequences. The
presence of Cuban physicians may decrease the workforce prepared to work
in the rural areas, introduce double standards in employment conditions
among professionals, and lower the quality of accessible health care (significant language barriers between the physicians, patients, and colleagues
may arise). The rapid changes in migration and professional registration
policy highlight the dynamic and complex nature of foreign recruitment—
a dynamic to which Nelson Mandela's presence has given a new twist.

Enter Mandela

Although the South African government has deliberately pursued policies that make it heavily dependent on migrant physicians, in 1997 Nelson
Mandela charted a very different course. During a visit to London, Mandela
issued a surprise plea to the UK government. Mobilizing his considerable
charisma and moral leverage, he pressed the British to ban the recruitment
of South African nurses. Mandela criticized Britain for recruiting nurses
from his country, which was facing a critical nursing shortage. Stop these recruitment campaigns, he urged, on humanitarian grounds. Mandela's re-

quest had a dramatic impact in the United Kingdom and also a ripple effect. It refueled the debate on the ethics of recruiting nurses from developing countries having already seriously reduced nursing workforces.

The first evidence of Mandela's powerful message was action within the United Kingdom. In 1999 the Department of Health in England responded with its first set of guidelines: "It is essential that all National Health Service employers do not actively recruit from developing countries which are experiencing nursing shortages of their own."[11] Highlighting the close link between Mandela's request and the development of these guidelines, South Africa was specifically mentioned as a country to avoid. But in all the emotional debate surrounding Mandela's statement and the subsequent British response, the fact that South Africa's health system continued to recruit and be dependent on migrant physicians was not widely publicized.

Mandela's call for an overseas ban on the recruitment of South African nurses was an effective political maneuver. By encouraging foreign governments to implement such a ban, Mandela attempted to avoid the kind of criticism he would have received at home if he had tried to prohibit nurses from leaving South Africa. This ploy did not fool South African nurses.

Even though the 1999 UK ban on recruitment in South Africa does not prevent nurses from responding directly to recruitment ads, South African nurses nevertheless considered this a violation of their human rights. The Democratic Nursing Organization of South Africa (DENOSA) journal carried an article that said: "The South African authorities must have been quite aware that should the ban have been introduced by the South African authorities it could easily be proved to be an infringement of the rights of the individual in terms of the South African Constitution and would surely have been found to be unconstitutional if challenged by South African nurses. But now that the ban has been introduced by a host country, it cannot be challenged in terms of South Africa's Constitution."[12]

The South African nurses also questioned the timing of this measure, which came very soon after a dramatic downsizing of the health sector. The DENOSA editor reported the significant unemployment of nurses and new graduates unable to find positions in the public sector.[13] At a time when nurses were unable to find work in South Africa, options to obtain employment abroad were diminishing.

Codes of Practice

The South African government's attempt to keep its nurses from emigrating found strong support, but from outside the country—again starting in the United Kingdom. This is particularly ironic because the United Kingdom is one of the industrialized countries that is most dependent on foreign nurse recruitment. Yet England was among the first to develop a code to reduce the practice.[14] Looking closely at the interplay between political action and inaction in England and South Africa, we gain an even better understanding of the powerful vested interests at stake. In this case, the players include employers desperate to relieve their staffing shortages, recruitment agencies with strong business incentives, and health professionals eager to find opportunities to substantially increase their earnings.[15]

All four countries that make up the United Kingdom—England, Scotland, Wales, and Northern Ireland—have their own national health services. The English National Health Service (NHS), however, employs 73 percent of all nurses and 90 percent of the international nurse recruits in the United Kingdom. In 1999 the Department of Health of England set an important precedent for the United Kingdom, and indeed for the Commonwealth, when it released its "Guidance on International Nursing Recruitment." The English action specifically required NHS employers to avoid active recruitment in South Africa and the Caribbean. In September 2001 the department released an even broader and more detailed "Code of Practice for NHS Employers Involved in the Recruitment of Healthcare Professionals." In 2003 it added other countries to a list of less-developed countries to be avoided. Private recruitment agencies were also invited to adhere to the code and become recognized as an approved agency. NHS employers were instructed to deal only with agencies on this list.

Although this so-called ban sounds draconian, it illustrates the difficulty of regulating, let alone restricting, nurse migration. The focus of these initiatives is the establishment of ethical practices. The 2003 guidelines are, however, voluntary, without formal legal basis, focus only on active recruitment, and are limited to government facilities within the National Health Service. No enforcement machinery was introduced, and independent or for-profit employers (a growing sector especially active in the care of older persons) as well as recruitment agencies remained beyond the scope of the guidelines.

Effectiveness of the code has been challenged on several fronts. Most criticism focuses on its voluntary nature and its narrow scope. The excluded private sector is, in fact, a backdoor entrance that allows migrant nurses access to the National Health Service where the pay, benefits, and working conditions tend to be better than those offered by private employers. Once nurses have been recruited and are working in the United Kingdom they have the right to change employers. The nurse Ethel Nkosi may therefore manage to bypass both South African protests and English "restrictions" by getting a job through the active recruitment of a private-sector nursing home in Manchester. Once she is in the job and becomes aware of the disparity in pay, she can easily switch to the public sector. If she takes this circuitous route, that she originally came from one of the source countries designated by the code no longer matters.

The polemic continues. As of April 1, 2004, the first ten NHS foundation trusts came into being. In the UK National Health Services, primary care trusts provide community care while hospital trusts provide acute health care. These trusts are free-standing statutory bodies responsible for their own budgets and priorities while being guided by the directives determined by the Strategic Health Authority or the Department of Health (DOH). According to the DOH, these newly introduced foundation trusts form part of a major program of investment, expansion, and reform of the National Health Service. While they continue to treat patients according to NHS principles and standards, the trusts are controlled and run locally. What has come as a surprise to many is the sudden exclusion of foundation trusts from the obligations of the DOH code of practice dealing with foreign recruitment of health professionals. UK unions reacted with "astonishment at the 'shameful' u-turn on poaching nurses from developing countries," reports Hélène Mulholland of the *Guardian*, "just two months after the health secretary, John Reid, pledged to strengthen the code of conduct on ethical recruitment."[16] Mulholland classifies this move as a quite unethical erosion of the code.

According to the senior employment relations adviser of the Royal College of Nursing, Howard Catton, "The competitive environment being encouraged in the health sector through 'payment by results,' was likely to encourage foundation hospitals to abandon the code to secure the staff necessary to deliver extra capacity."[17] The fact that statistics prove that the ban has had no significant effect on foreign nurse recruitment from developing countries is not discussed. Even the weak attempts to remedy problems have once again been compromised by vested interests, and the fundamental reasons for the mass migration continue to be neglected. Though the measure provides no more than a false sense of security, everyone—including the very ministers who decided to narrow the recruitment code's scope—seems to publicly defend it. Perhaps they believe that to be seen promoting a strategy, even an ineffective one, is better than having no strategy at all. If so, this belief begs some reflection.

The distinction between active and passive recruitment adds to the confusion and allows migration to continue relatively unabated. The code says that the NHS cannot engage in active recruitment of nurses in prohibited countries. So when the NHS or one of its facilities places an ad in a nursing journal or newspaper, or posts a vacancy notice on the Internet where anyone can read it, is this passive or active recruitment? Does the end result really differ? What is aggressive recruitment? How are these terms defined? Some use quantity to define the qualitative term *aggressive*. If a recruitment agency recruits a hundred nurses at one time from a given country, this may be considered an act of aggressive recruitment. But is it aggressive if ten agencies recruit ten nurses each, or fifty agencies recruit two nurses each? If an agency recruits one specialist nurse, but the only one in a given province or country, should this be considered aggressive recruitment? Giving different definitions to processes that lead to the same ends cannot solve the ethical problems embedded in foreign recruitment. Obviously, much is left to the imagination of those involved in the recruitment process and interpretations may vary, but the realities are unchanged: Britain remains dependent on foreign nurses, and they are usually supplied by countries considered to be unethical sources of recruitment.

James Buchan and Julie Sochalski argue that codes are weakened by the "inadequacy of information systems needed for policy analysis and decision-making."[18] International monitoring of migration is almost impossible without reliable workforce data at the national level. Such data would provide a clear overview of how many nurses there are in a particular country, what percentage are working in the country's health sector (public and private), what positions are filled, and how many nurses are going abroad and where. Given that chronic concern over nurse shortages and "brain drain" has been expressed since the 1970s, one might think governments would have introduced effective data collection mechanisms over the last thirty years. Most have, however, lacked the political will to finance the establishment of effective information systems. For example, the Commonwealth, while agreeing that workforce planning is of paramount importance, recognizes that this fundamental management process is often absent and seriously hampered by inadequate data when it actually takes place.[19]

In addition to basic workforce planning information, data on how nurses arrive in the destination country are essential when evaluating the impact of ethical recruitment codes. At present no country can accurately provide this information. They do not seem to be able to carefully chart the routes to employment, how they are traveled, and who travels along them. This in spite of the fact that we know the various ways nurses make their way to employment in another country. Yet from the current statistics that are routinely gathered, it is impossible to identify whether people have been actively recruited or have made individual applications.[20] In order to evaluate the impact of ethical recruitment codes this basic information is essential. Not only have sanctions and incentives not been incorporated in the codes but concrete measures to evaluate their impact have been neglected. The UK data actually available indicate that only one-third of migrant nurses are recruited by agencies. The great majority find their way to Britain by other means, and yet the political focus continues to be on recruitment agencies.

The code has failed to encourage recruitment agencies to adhere to its principles and apply for agency approval. Yet, recruitment agencies had a significant incentive to do both. Approved agencies would attract a bigger share of the post-code market. Relatively few agencies, however, made the effort (68 out of approximately 115). One of the reasons many agencies gave for their lack of interest in applying was their belief that the code's selection criterion was impossible to satisfy. In a bureaucratic Catch-22, agencies are "only eligible to be on the Department of Health's list of approved agencies if they obtain two references from NHS trusts verifying that they adhere to the code of practice. This can create difficulties because they cannot gain access to the approved list unless they have references from the NHS, and NHS managers will not use an agency that is not on the approved list."[21] In fact, only agencies that had been dealing with NHS managers and were already following the recommended practices could obtain the necessary references to get on the list. Take the situation of an agency that in the past was not recruiting "ethically" but wanted to change its practices so that it could get on the list. How would the agency be able to get the necessary references since NHS managers were not allowed to work with them?

There is no evidence at this time that the DOH guidelines are effective in reducing the active recruitment from developing countries that have nursing shortages of their own. While there appears to have been a short-term impact on reducing the numbers of nurses that came from South Africa and the Caribbean in 1999, recruitment from other source countries actually accelerated. Two years after the code was released, the level of recruitment from South Africa once again increased to its previous rate.[22] Although they were on the list of developing countries to be avoided, in 2003 annual recruitment of nurses from Ghana, Nigeria, and Zimbabwe to England managed to increase.[23] Indeed, one in three work permits issued to nurses involved applicants from countries where active recruitment is prohibited.

Paul Burstow, a Liberal Democrat member of Parliament, called the Department of Health's code a sham. "The government's whole approach of dealing with international recruitment is really window dressing, designed to give confidence that nurses will not be exploited and abused, when in practice that is exactly what is happening for too many of them when they come."[24] Indeed, the Department of Health again came under fire when, under pressure to reduce waiting lists for hip and knee surgery, it seemed to abandon its own principles and signed contracts to bring Netcare South African nurses on short-term contracts to help meet its targeted waiting list reductions. According to the editor of *Nursing Times*, "The DoH's defense is that the nurses come from South Africa's independent sector. This is disingenuous. The South African independent sector creams off the best nurses from an understaffed workforce that is trying hard to provide care to the poorest in society. The gap left by nurses leaving the sector can only be filled by turning to those who are treating the most needy. . . . It is no good the DoH fingerwagging at the independent sector in the UK for flouting its ethical recruitment guidance, only to lead by bad example when it suits."[25]

The Netcare contracts are another example of how protecting nurses and patients founders on the shoals of political imperatives. Nelson Mandela, who pressed the United Kingdom to ban the recruitment of South African nurses, has supported Netcare's efforts to provide it with temporary nurses. The migration of South African nurses to the United Kingdom seems to be encouraged if nurses are brought in on a temporary basis. But by introducing more complex issues and double standards with regard to these nurses' qualification assessments and registration, the new contracts clearly send mixed messages to the whole health system.

Nurses who work in the United Kingdom are supposed to be registered in one of the four countries—England, Scotland, Wales, or Northern Ireland. In many cases, they must also work through an adaptation period with three to nine months and sometimes more of supervised practice. Will these temporary nurses be required to register in the United Kingdom? How will the Netcare nurses meet the adaptation period requirements if their contract is for three months only? Bending the rules to accommodate a political priority, namely, shorter waiting lists, may pose problems of another order.

If we use England as a case study of attempts to ethically regulate nurse migration, we find that this effort seems to have produced more questions than functioning models. Two major queries emerge. First, why spend the time, finances, and energy to develop a code that will not be seriously enforced or effectively evaluated? Second, is this merely an example of gesture politics—a lip-service public campaign exercise that responds to expressed humanitarian concerns while allowing the disputed international flow of nurses from developing countries to continue? Even more questions are raised when we examine how the UK exercise served as the impetus for the development of a code of practice for the nations in the British Commonwealth.

The Commonwealth Code of Practice

When England developed its code, it did not apply to nurses recruited to health systems in Northern Ireland, Wales, or Scotland or any other Commonwealth country. It did, however, serve as an inspiration throughout the United Kingdom and for the other fifty-one countries in the Commonwealth.

Apparently ignoring the lack of evidence with regard to the effectiveness of the English code, and discounting the many criticisms of its implementation, the Commonwealth secretariat decided to develop its very own— slightly improved but very similar—code of practice. With much fanfare, the Commonwealth adopted the Code of Practice for the International Recruitment of Health Workers in May 2003. Even though signing on to the Commonwealth code is a formality since it is not a binding document, only twenty-two Commonwealth nations enlisted as signatories, perhaps a sign of the conflict of interest between different pressure groups at home. Not surprisingly, all but one of the twenty-two signatories are developing countries, nations that have the most to gain from its application. In 2004 a series of regional workshops was given to present the code, raise awareness of the issues, and consider strategies to address staff shortages in the health sector. Member countries and Commonwealth migration experts recognized that the focus needs to be broader than just preventing health professionals from migrating.

The code upholds the right of health workers to migrate in pursuit of a range of advantages and serves to safeguard the potential benefits that migration can bring. In other words, the Commonwealth recognizes that individuals have the right to leave their country and that migration can benefit all concerned, under the right conditions. Two further key points are emphasized. First, the code stresses national sovereignty with regard to professional regulation and registration. Each country therefore continues to determine the education and practice requirements of persons granted the right to practice a given profession. The second point focuses on the responsibility of member countries to retain their trained personnel, an interesting and extremely innovative approach.[26] Once again, however, the code is not a legal document and provides no enforcement machinery to support its application.

The guiding principles are transparency, fairness, and mutuality of benefits. The code introduces the concepts of compensation, reparation, or restitution, three strategies the destination country can use to reciprocate for the advantages gained from the source country. By stipulating these mechanisms, the code recognizes the complex bargains and trade-offs that are at the heart of migration.

The permanent emigration of a health professional represents a loss, not only of skills to the health sector of the source country, but also of the country's investment in the health professional's education at the primary and secondary as well as tertiary levels. Taking Ghana as an example, experts estimate tuition costs conservatively at $20,000 per medical student. During the ten-year period 1985–94, the expense of educating graduates from the country's medical and nursing schools, who have now emigrated, represents an overall loss of $10–15 million. "Such financial losses are occurring in countries least able to afford them and which do not have the resources to effectively tackle their problems of migration."[27]

In many cases it is true that recruiting foreign-educated nurses may be a cost-saving measure for the destination country—one that comes at the expense of education budgets of poorer countries. But that is not always the case. The tertiary or nursing-school education of the migrant nurse is not always an expense of the source country's government. Increasingly, nursing education is privately funded, even in some poorer countries like the Philippines. Similarly, destination countries do not always save on education costs of homegrown nurses when they employ foreign ones. That is because private education is becoming much more common in industrialized countries that used to depend almost exclusively on publicly funded educational systems. In a sense, different "pockets" are involved in covering the cost, and direct monetary compensation becomes a very complex exercise as the number of different parties directly concerned increases.

The Commonwealth code of practice proposes compensation in the form of technical or financial assistance, training programs, or the facilitation of the migrant worker's return to the source country if applicable. But here again, the critical issue of return migration bumps into numerous conflicts and contradictions. Ideally, return migration should be the responsibility of both the destination and source country. If a country is suffering from a nursing shortage, it would seem logical that it would want its migrant nurses to return quickly. While many source countries say they are desperately concerned that their nurses are leaving, strangely enough, as we learned from the stories of migrant nurses presented earlier, strategies to facilitate their return are for the most part absent.

One of the key mechanisms that would encourage migrating nurses to return to their country would be policies that allow them long-term leaves of absences from their places of employment. Many nurses in developing countries work for publicly funded and government-run hospitals. These governments, unlike those in countries where hospitals are privately run, have a great deal of control over the reemployment of the migrant. But many migrant nurses in such systems say that their governments staunchly refuse to encourage such reemployment policies.

Frequently, health systems do not acknowledge professional accomplishments and the advanced skills and knowledge acquired from experience abroad. In fact, if migrant nurses were to return from abroad, they would not get a promotion; they would probably be demoted. Migrant nurses considering a return to their home country usually face moving into a position offering a lower salary, with less responsibility, and requiring fewer skills. Thus a nurse who has acquired more education, more skill, and more experience is actually penalized.

Many health services refuse to allow leave without pay because they erroneously believe that their refusal will dissuade nurses from migrating. A country's strategy to retain its nurses in active practice must, however, accept the reality that migration will tend to increase in this globalized world. It is in the country's interest to have these migrant nurses return home to useful employment, taking full advantage of the skills and knowledge acquired abroad. Policies introduced to discourage initial migration may be an obstacle to nurses' return and ultimately prove counterproductive. Starting in 2005, the Department of Health of Gauteng (South Africa) is making available a two-year leave of absence for nurses who wish to work abroad and then return to a secure post with no loss of benefits. This initiative is worth monitoring closely. If effective, it will encourage brain circulation, improve family revenues, and decrease brain drain.

The code's legitimate efforts to assure national sovereignty in regulation and registration and to determine education and practice requirements highlights the complex nature of international mobility. It is important that the standards of care in any given country not be compromised and that all individuals practicing the profession meet at least the minimum standards of education and practice set in that country. For nursing, this point is critical if the profession's concerns for patient safety and guarantees for the protection of the title of nurse are to be respected. People who have not met the criteria will be prevented from holding nurse positions and taking on nurses' responsibilities. Patients, colleagues, and supervisors can feel safe knowing that the level of professional knowledge and skills expected from the registered nurse is guaranteed. Any code of ethics should assure this basic respect for the profession's integrity.

While the harmonization of education programs is beginning, there is still a long way to go before the worldwide recognition of nursing qualifications is automatic. In maintaining national sovereignty in the regulation of health professionals, the code recognizes the contemporary global realities without discouraging the development of mutual recognition agreements (to be discussed later).

The code insists on the responsibility of member countries, including developing countries, to retain their trained personnel. This critical element of retention needs to be emphasized when considering nurse migration, yet is often neglected in practice. In most countries too much attention is given to recruitment and not enough to retention. There is no point in recruiting a professional into a dysfunctional system, one that is unable to keep its workers in active practice. The whole exercise becomes a futile, endlessly repeating cycle that only aggravates the shortage, since it wastes available resources. It is in the interest of countries to retain a critical mass of qualified and actively practicing nurses to provide care and sustain the effective functioning of the health system.

Some politicians and health policy makers have argued that nurses working in impoverished developing countries cannot possibly receive the same salaries as those offered in richer, industrialized countries. As a result policies have attempted to restrict migration instead of providing better pay and working conditions locally. Most nurses, however, are reluctant to leave their home countries and would be quite willing to stay if offered a living wage. For example, in 2004 nurse emigration from Fiji was greatly reduced. When Fijian nurses learned that their government might soon reclassify their profession in the public-sector pay scale, thus improving their remuneration and access to a competitive wage, nurses postponed their decision to migrate. Relative income within home countries is critical. "Nurses are not asking for Australian and New Zealand salaries," says Kuini Lutua, chief executive officer of the Fiji Nurses Association. "If offered a decent wage and a safe work environment, nurses will stay in Fiji."

The Ministry of Health in Malawi is said to be facing the possible collapse of the health system due to the shortage of nurses willing to work. The ministry is proposing an increase in the number of nurses being trained while more than doubling their pay. According to recent interviews held in Lilongwe, "registered nurses, who make about $1,900 a year, said if their pay were doubled or tripled, they would be more likely to stay, but added that they had heard such promises before."[28]

Gender Implications

No consideration of efforts to deal with skilled migration are complete without considering the gender implications and inequalities embedded in this debate. Guidelines that masquerade as gender neutral may in fact be gender rigged and ranked. As Peggy Vidot, chief program officer for health at the Commonwealth secretariat, points out, although the Commonwealth code is meant to deal with all health professionals, discussions for the most part focus on the recruitment of nurses. In a similar move in 2001, health ministers of the Southern African Development Community (SADC) issued a statement titled "Recruitment of Health Personnel by Developed Countries."[29] Yet the very first paragraph specifically mentions and elaborates on the migration of nurses. There is a clear message that while international health-sector codes and statements on the migration of health personnel appear generic in nature, concern for an accessible nursing workforce is now a mobilizing force.

Research indicates that 75 percent of all classifications/grades are sex-segregated. In other words, there is a predominance of 70 percent or more of one gender in the classification, grade, or profession. The International Labour Organization has repeatedly confirmed that the relative value and degree of remuneration attributed to a certain occupation still seems to be influenced by the predominance of women in that occupation. In fact, comparable worth studies have shown that, on average, female-dominated jobs are paid 15 percent less than male-dominated jobs that require comparable levels of skills, effort, and responsibility.[30] For decades the nursing profession has suffered from a generalized discrimination in the workplace. This has led the International Council of Nurses to conclude that current salary structures are often based on gender and not on the value of the job to society.[31] Realizing that remuneration policies are gender biased, it may be said that the same discriminatory forces are at play in immigration/emigration policies. Governments and international organizations proclaim to all who will listen that they recognize the high value of nurses' contributions. Yet they simultaneously refuse to provide or promote competitive salaries and restrict their liberties.

Nurse migration is largely a female affair. One of its most positive aspects is the fact that it gives women a greater sense of independence and accomplishment. In her work on the history of nursing, Sioban Nelson argues that nursing has always been a perfect vehicle for this kind of female emancipation.[32] The fact that nursing has been so often viewed as a calling not a career, that it has been painted as self-sacrifice not self-fulfillment, that nurses have been forced to hide—and sometimes choose to hide—behind male/physician accomplishment has made it a perfect vehicle for traditional women to enter into previously prohibited public spaces, says Suzanne Gordon.[33]

Many observers have argued that this use of traditional feminine stereotypes and motifs also puts nurses in a peculiar professional position. Nurses, as women, seem to be singled out because their services are so essential and, at the same time, taken for granted. One has to ask, is it because they are women that the gender implications of these codes are ignored? Indeed, this question becomes even more pressing when one considers another step in the complexity of nurse migration, the emigration ban. Is it because they are women that nations are willing to ignore nurses' basic human right—the right to leave their country?

Emigration Bans

Article 13 (2) of the Universal Declaration of Human Rights adopted in 1948 by the United Nations gives everyone the right to leave their home country. There is no corresponding right of entry to another country. This is left to the immigration policy of individual destination countries. The right to leave, however, is a basic principle generally upheld in all the codes of practice and ethical recruitment guidelines.

Amazingly, when it comes to nurses, the introduction of emigration bans has become a persistent theme of the international regulatory agenda. Of course, policy makers argue that this is an indication of how critical the access to nurses has become. These bans, they insist, try to address pressing social problems by limiting or preventing nurses from leaving home countries that either face a critical nurse shortage or are convinced that their citizens are being victimized abroad.

Nurses, however, do not tend to view this strategy as one that either values or protects them. They view it for what it is—a violation of human rights.

Nurses worry about such bans because some nations have already initiated them. In 1998 Bangladesh introduced a travel ban on women wishing to work abroad. The given rationale was that migrant women were particularly vulnerable to abuse and were badly treated abroad. National human rights and women's organizations, including the Bangladesh Women Lawyers' Association, strongly criticized this policy, pointing out that the government "must look beyond bans as a protective mechanism and look at briefing and empowering migrant workers before they leave the country and respond to their needs while overseas."[34]

The government has since lifted the restriction on female nurses working abroad but has maintained the ban on domestic workers, the nature of whose work (in private homes) makes monitoring of abuses difficult.[35] Bangladesh in April 2003 decided to relax even these latest restrictions, but only for women workers over thirty-five accompanying their husbands abroad for work.

Despite the official ban, it is estimated that fifty thousand Bangladeshi women have left the country since it was imposed. Labor recruitment agents say that restrictions on the export of female workers are not very effective— a total ban cannot be enforced and only encourages irregular migration. An anonymous official at the Bureau of Manpower, Employment and Training explained that, since the ban was introduced, Bangladeshis have been taking advantage of a loophole in the law that allows women to leave the country if accompanied by their husbands or brothers. Dishonest recruitment agencies were sending women abroad with forged passports and false marriage registration certificates.[36]

Financial gain may be the reason why the ban has been so poorly enforced. Overseas workers sent more than $2 billion back to Bangladesh in the form of remittances. According to Tabibul Islam, authorities are hoping that with the relaxation of the present ban an additional one hundred thousand women workers per year will be employed overseas, the clear motivation being an increase in the remittances received.

In fact, the government's vested interests in the form of remittances have generated a change in attitude and policy with regard to emigration bans. Yet, nothing seems to have been done to ensure that these migrant women are better protected. The empowerment programs recommended by human rights and women's groups have not been implemented. Bilateral negotiations with destination countries are only beginning, although the bans are already being relaxed. While women should rejoice that the oppressive measure is being lifted, they should be concerned that the risks to their personal safety are still present. This puts into question the justification for the bans in the first place.

As we have seen, the two earliest and most widely known recruitment bans were developed in England and Ireland (1999 and 2001 respectively). It is important to recall that as their names indicate—"DOH Guidance on International Nursing Recruitment" and "DOHC Guidance for Best Practice on the Recruitment of Overseas Nurses and Midwives"—these documents focused completely on nurses. It was only later that other health professionals were incorporated in the code of practice for England and the one developed by the Commonwealth.

It seems clear that gender is a dominant force in the creation and focus of these bans. Other professions, for example, physicians and information technologists, have experienced high global demand within the international labor market. And yet no significant attempt has been made to curb the export potential of these predominantly male professionals although the need in many of the source countries was just as great as for nurses today.

Editorials in medical journals have repeatedly called for an ethical recruitment code for physicians. No serious proposal has ever appeared. The World Medical Association (WMA) waited until 2003 to issue its ethical guidelines for the international recruitment of physicians.[37]

The WMA guidelines recommend that countries recruiting physicians from another country should do so only in terms of and in accordance with the provisions of a memorandum of understanding between the countries. These guidelines present the professionals' perspective on a critical issue but impose no legal obligation on governments or physicians. Since they refer to government-to-government recruitment, much of the health labor market is exempt from this approach because many physicians work in the private sector and with individual employers. The guidelines also specifically state that physicians should not be prevented from leaving their home or adopted country to pursue career opportunities in another country.

We have seen that migration depends on access to information and at times financial support. As this is often provided by recruitment agencies, it can be argued that the deliberate absence of, or ban on, recruitment agency activity (for example, supplying job information, supporting the migration process, or providing relocation assistance) may constitute a direct obstacle to career opportunities abroad. Physicians defend their right to work abroad and this right has not been seriously challenged anywhere.

The other profession that has attracted attention when it comes to international recruitment is teaching. A working group met in February 2004 to develop ethical codes of conduct for the recruitment of teachers in the Commonwealth.[38] Senior officials considered the degree to which present practices afford sufficient protection to countries that have invested heavily in teacher training and to teachers recruited for service abroad.

As mentioned, the ILO has argued that the relative value and level of remuneration attributed to a certain occupation is heavily influenced by the predominance of women in that occupation. Did the chronic underinvestment of employers and governments in nursing (lower salaries, poor working conditions, inadequate staffing levels, reduced number of training positions) and the lack of recognition for nurses' contribution to patient well-being globally create professionals particularly vulnerable to the (real and false) promises of international recruitment agencies? Was nursing, a predominantly female profession, considered by policy makers and government authorities to be easier to manipulate or exploit? Ethical recruitment instruments are of too recent origin for any research conclusions as to the sociological environment facilitating their development and the implications of their attempted application. These are all questions that need to be raised, but for the moment no definitive answer is available.

Vested interests, inconsistencies, and double standards all play a major role and exert significant forces on the worldwide migration of nurses. International policies, agreements, and rules have a strong, direct impact on our daily lives in this era of rapid globalization. Bilateral and multilateral trade agreements promise economic development and facilitate international migration, but what will the future bring? What interests will predominate in the discussions and policy making? Will inequalities be allowed to persist? The regulation of international trade in professional services, often negotiated behind closed doors, is an arena where powerful vested interests are on display.

5. Trade and Migration

Denise Duvoisin, born in Europe and educated in the United States, is now registered to practice in Switzerland as a generalist nurse. She works in a Swiss clinic owned by a US-based private chain of hospitals. Duvoisin plays a key role within a multinational team of health professionals. Her patients are for the most part from Eastern Europe, unfamiliar with the local language and customs. Today, she bends over her postoperative patient, concerned that she cannot communicate with him. Although both nurse and patient are multilingual, they do not share a common language.

The cardiovascular surgery was successful and the patient's arteries are clear and bringing an unimpeded stream of blood to his heart. The danger of a heart attack has been averted, but Duvoisin is now concerned about preventing a common postoperative complication, pneumonia. Respiratory therapy has been ordered. Duvoisin needs to help the patient breathe deeply and cough, thus removing secretions lying deep at the bottom of his lungs— a painful process creating great pressures on the dozens of surgical stitches that lie all along the sternum. Duvoisin knows that coughing, which is normally so simple and taken for granted, is in this instance a life-saving measure that costs the patient much suffering. It is critical that she explain this to her patient. But language is proving a difficult barrier.

Duvoisin is also worried about an additional obstacle to her patient's recovery. A rare bacterium has been isolated in the patient's sputum culture and a specialist was contacted. The consultant, based in a foreign country, depends on sophisticated information technology to receive the vital baseline data, undertake the rapid analysis, and participate in the subsequent treatment planning of his colleagues. The team in Switzerland waits for the faxed laboratory results and phone consultation.

The case above is a typical postoperative scenario today. Twenty years ago, when this actually took place, truly multinational health professional teams treating a foreigner in Switzerland, with the help of laboratories and specialists in the United States, was exceptional. What allows all this to occur routinely now is largely the result of international trade and migration.

Previous chapters have shown how migration has created numerous opportunities for businesses all over the world and how countries have tried to regulate this trade and address the multiple ethical issues that arise. If setting a framework for immigration is difficult at a national and regional level, the complexity escalates when the word *international* refers to the global economy in which hundreds of nations, hundreds of thousands of businesses, and millions of workers participate.

The very existence of businesses and institutions involved in international trade depends on a global structure of rules and regulations, negotiations, and agreements. The professional and personal lives of the nurses who work for them—and in a sense the fate of the nursing profession and the patients it serves—hang in the balance. This is where multilateral trade agreements (MTAs), regional trade agreements (RTAs), bilateral trade agreements (BTAs), or international trade agreements (ITAs) and the General Agreement on Trade in Services (GATS) of the World Trade Organization enter the picture.

Whether we are aware of them or not, whether we understand the implications of the manifold statements and exceptions or remain bewildered, international trade agreements regulate this rapidly expanding market activity. They define the rules of commercial transactions between nations and facilitate the creation of an international marketplace.

Yet those who try to understand the economic underpinnings of this new marketplace confront an enormous challenge. They have to plow through long and tedious texts, full of complex legal language laced with technical jargon and multiple exceptions in small print to almost every rule. One North American trade agreement has been jokingly described as "2000 pages of what governments can no longer do."[1] For the uninitiated, these agreements are, to put it mildly, laborious reading.

Take this excerpt from article 27 of GATS: "A member may deny the benefits of this Agreement to the supply of a service, if it establishes that the service is supplied from or in the territory of a non-Member or of a Member to which the denying Member does not apply the WTO Agreement."[2] This example may convince you that reading ITAs is best avoided. The cost of ignoring the content of these global agreements is, however, increasingly high. Neglecting trade agreements is no longer an affordable option.

To do so allows others to decide the rules for how we live our lives. This presents a great personal and societal risk, which is why around the world thousands of people—and not just political activists—plunge into the arena of global trade and try to understand its ground rules, negotiations, and implications. According to Susan Aaronson, "a wide range of citizens has become concerned about the effect of trade rules upon the achievement of other important policy goals. In India, Latin America, Europe, Canada and the United States, alarmed citizens have taken to the streets to protest globalization and in particular what they perceive as the undemocratic nature" of trade negotiations.[3] Their concerns have produced massive and very passionate, sometimes violent, public demonstrations at recent ministerial conferences of the World Trade Organization (WTO) and the World Economic Forum. This is proof that more and more people are aware of the potential power of trade agreements, intend to voice their opinion publicly, and wish to influence the negotiation outcomes by whatever means are necessary.

Much of the reporting on these discussions and protests concerns traditional manufacturing and agricultural products—like farming subsidies, tariffs placed on imported steel, or the market access of bananas. ITAs have traditionally focused on the trade of goods and commodities, the reduction of tariffs, and the opening of national markets to foreign imports such as bananas, steel, or pharmaceuticals. The prime example of an ITA is the famous multilateral GATT (General Agreement on Tariffs and Trade), established by negotiations among the Western industrialized nations after World War II.

Human services, however, are now also on the negotiating table. Global trade agreements will decide who takes care of us when we are in hospital, just as they already determine whether we eat genetically modified foods, whether we have access to cheaper generic drugs, or whether workers see their factories close down due to competition from abroad. ITAs may now seek to reduce trade barriers and promote the mobility of services and persons as well as capital and goods. Although relatively new, the concept of international trade in services is a key component of the globalization landscape.

Trade in Services

Services are often defined as goods that are produced and consumed simultaneously. They usually have a direct impact on or change the consumer in some way: a haircut enhances a person's appearance, swimming lessons impart a new skill, and surgery removes an infected appendix, for example.[4] As a current and future source of economic growth (or profit) for individuals, enterprises and nations, the services sector is generating great interest in the global marketplace.

The generally low level of international trade in services in the past has been attributed to three factors. First, institutional, administrative, or technical constraints, such as the existence of public-sector monopolies in education and telephone services, have discouraged trade initiatives. Second, strict access regulations and controls in financial investment and various professional services have also reduced certain trade opportunities. Lastly, the need for direct physical contact between suppliers and consumers (i.e., caregivers and patients or teachers and students), a fundamental characteristic of health and social services up to now, was considered to be an insurmountable obstacle.[5] Recently, however, many of these barriers have either diminished or completely disappeared, creating an environment that is more conducive to this innovative type of international trade.

As a sector, services represent a major and growing share of employment and production in countries worldwide. The trade in all kinds of services—from health care to information technology, banking, or tourism—is expected to continue to expand faster than the trade in goods. Already, turnover or sales in the services sector in the United States and Luxembourg is around 3.5 times higher than in the manufacturing sector. Services are now the major economic sector in OECD countries, accounting for 50–70 percent of industrial activity or gross domestic product.[6] Job creation in services is exceeding overall job growth in OECD countries, with about 65 percent of workers employed in this sector.[7] Looking at worldwide figures, the WTO estimates that "services currently account for over 60% of global production and employment."[8]

The implementation of the General Agreement on Trade in Services (GATS) in 1995 is considered a milestone in the history of the multilateral trading system. Ever since the Second World War, industrial nations tried to both expand and regulate international commerce. In the 1940s the United States and Britain initiated the negotiations that finally established the International Trade Organization (ITO) and the General Agreement on Tariffs and Trade (GATT), which helped establish a framework to both govern and promote global commerce. GATT, which was meant to be a temporary multilateral agreement, provided nations with a set of rules and a forum to negotiate reductions in barriers to trade.

The ITO was an international institution and seat for a code of world trade principles. According to Aaronson, "The ITO represented an internationalization of the view that governments could play a positive role in encouraging international economic growth. It was incredibly comprehensive: including chapters on commercial policy, investment, employment and even business practices (what we call antitrust or competition policies today)."[9] The ITO was never popular, however. Leading nations, including the

United States, never brought ITO membership before their legislatures for a vote, so this body was doomed. Consequently, the provisional GATT governed world trade until 1994.

After the establishment of GATT, participating nations held eight round-table talks on the reduction of trade barriers. Business and political interests in many nations began pushing for a more binding legal framework in which trade barriers could be reduced, trade expanded, and disputes settled. They encouraged action to formalize GATT and create a much more powerful international trade organization. This pressure bore fruit in what is commonly called the Uruguay Round of trade talks held from 1986 to 1993. The Uruguay Round ultimately led to the creation of the World Trade Organization. Replacing and greatly expanding the purview of the GATT secretariat, the WTO holds greater reach and power to oversee the function of trade agreements (including specific agreements for goods, services, intellectual property, and the settlement of trade disputes) and acts as a permanent forum for trade negotiations and rule making.[10]

While GATT regulates the trade in goods, GATS plays this fundamental role for the trade in services. In concept, GATS is the most far-reaching and enforceable agreement addressing such trade. It is a multilateral framework for regulating international trade in services and applies to all WTO members (147 countries as of April 2004). This document underscores the importance governments and policy makers assign to the service sector as a potential source of future economic development in industrialized as well as developing countries. Since February 2000, negotiations have been underway in the WTO to expand and "fine-tune" GATS.

The agreement has "a wide scope and applies to all services supplied on a commercial basis. It excludes most air transport as well as services supplied in the exercise of governmental authority (defined as service supplied neither on a commercial basis nor in competition with one or more service suppliers)."[11] Typical examples of the latter include police, fire protection, monetary policy operations, mandatory social security, and tax and customs administration.

GATS has three objectives. First, to progressively liberalize trade in services through successive rounds of negotiations. Second, to encourage economic growth and development through the liberalization of trade in services—essentially reducing trade barriers and opening national markets to foreign enterprises, capital, or workers. And last, to increase the participation of developing countries in world trade in services. The agreement consists of two fundamental parts. Like the architects of a new global chess game, GATS designs the board, prepares the players, provides the rules, and determines the legitimate moves as well as the penalties. Part 1 elaborates a series of rules that define general obligations for the signatories, while part 2 establishes a framework under which countries declare which service sectors foreign suppliers will be allowed to enter and under what conditions. These are called "specific commitments." For the purposes of clarity, a list of 12 service sectors and approximately 160 subsectors are made available. The main service sectors include business services, communication services, construction and related engineering services, distribution services, educational services, environmental services, financial services, health-related and social services, tourism and travel-related services, transport services, and recreational, cultural and sporting services. It is possible to consult the services commitments of WTO members on the WTO website, which indicates market access conditions and limitations. GATS sets out four possible modes or ways in which services can be traded between WTO members.[12]

The GATS definition of trade in services "emerged from a grand North-South bargain: when industrial countries sought the inclusion of investment in services, developing countries insisted on a symmetrical treatment of all factor movements—that is, parity between capital and labor."[13] In other words, industrial countries with funds or capital wanted to open new markets as a type of financial investment. This would facilitate business or corporate expansion, either by establishing a new business in another country or creating a new branch of a transnational corporation, usually based in an industrialized country. Developing countries, with limited financial resources, were less interested in such an option and more concerned about finding employment for their citizens, who are often unemployed or underemployed. Negotiations were concluded and both these dimensions of international trade in services—the movement of capital and the movement of labor—now appear in the final text.

Modes of Supply in the Trade of Health Services

As we have seen, health care is among the most rapidly growing sectors in the world economy today. It generates an estimated $3 trillion per year in the OECD countries alone, and this figure is expected to rise to $4 trillion by 2005.[14] Trade in health services is considered minimal when compared to other traded services, for example, tourism and information technology. Nevertheless, as health services are liberalized, entry barriers are lowered, and technology is developed, the prediction is that the trade in health services will rapidly increase.

Services are delivered and traded in various ways. And here is where the language gets really interesting. According to GATS, the supply of a service includes its production, distribution, marketing, sale, and delivery. The "service supplier" is any person that supplies a service and a distinction is made between "natural person" and "juridical person." A "natural person" is a national or permanent resident of a given country. A "juridical person" means any legal entity duly constituted or otherwise organized under applicable law.[15] So Nurse Duvoisin, whose case set the scene for this chapter, is granted the status of a "natural person," while the transnational company that owns and runs the facility—her employer—is a "juridical person."

Mention the term "natural person" and it generates two contradictory reactions. The legalese can dull readers' and policy makers' sensitivity to the fact that the articles in GATS actually deal with the fate of human beings and their families. Or the term can produce a high-voltage shock, fixing one's attention on the very human dimension of trade agreements.

Although recently developed, the GATS classification with its four modes of supply is widely applied to characterize and compare trade agreements. To understand the new world of nurse migration, it is useful to explore each category in more depth.

Using the GATS labels, mode 1 refers to *cross-border supply:* a service supplied from the territory of one WTO member into the territory of any other WTO member. For the health sector, this includes the shipment by traditional mail services of laboratory samples and clinical consultation. With the introduction of information technology, it now also incorporates the electronic delivery of test results, diagnoses, and advice. Either migrant or homegrown nurses may thus be interpreting test results that have been established by a laboratory based in a different country and communicated by phone, fax, traditional mail, or e-mail. In fact, mode 1 will apply to more and more nurses because of the increased use of telemedicine and telenursing. Recently, an urgent request from Tanzania was sent to a web-based WHO chat room. The surgeon from Sengerema District Hospital pleaded for urgent professional advice from colleagues around the world to deal with his patient, a newly born baby delivered with its entire heart and intestines outside its body. The call for specialists was made by e-mail and sent worldwide in an instant.[16] Electronic consultation will become increasingly common as health care providers and patients have easier access to computers and the Internet.

Today it is possible for a clinician in one country to treat and monitor a patient in another through a variety of telehealth services. Telehealth is defined as the delivery of health care and health care–related services through the use of telecommunications technologies.[17] These begin with basic telephone service (known as the plain old telephone service, or POTS, to distinguish it from the more complex technologies that have emerged in recent times) and now integrate radio, video, and computer technology. All types of health disciplines use advanced technology, including telepathology, teleradiology, telepsychiatry and telenursing. Here is how D. Milholland describes a common telehealth scenario:

> In a US city, individuals requiring complex intravenous fluids, medications and feeding, and physiological monitoring can be managed in their homes via a combination of electronic and in-person nursing visits. During the electronic visits, a two-way, interactive video-based telephone system is used. The nurse at the distant base can observe both overall appearance and function and, through a special lens, can examine wounds and intravenous sites. The nurse and the client can speak directly to each other. Physiological monitoring data can be collected automatically and transmitted to the nurse.[18]

While this example is domestic—the nurse provides care at a distance but from within the same country—international cases are increasing. Many cross-border telemedicine initiatives have emerged. US hospitals provide their counterparts in Central America and the eastern Mediterranean with telediagnostic, surveillance, and consultation services. Telediagnosis services are also provided by hospitals in China's coastal provinces to patients in Macao, Taiwan, and some Southeast Asian countries.[19] Global demand for telehealth services is estimated at $1.25 trillion annually, which includes direct clinical services, professional backup services, consumer health information–related services, continuing professional education services, and management of health care delivery services.[20]

Definitions of nursing practice and accountability change dramatically when technology makes it possible for companies or professionals to provide cross-border services. But it creates as many problems as it solves. If patients in one country have access to health services from another country, this gives rise to concerns about quality assurance, practice oversight, and control over the qualifications of those providing the services. The ethical and legal liability questions that emerge are beginning to attract more attention. A functional regulatory framework will need to be established to ensure accountability for professional practice as well as patient safety before this booming business will be internationally creditable.

Although the delivery of a service by a nurse in one country to a patient in another may not seem directly related to international nurse migration, in fact telenursing represents a "virtual" mobility that raises many of the same issues. Do professional registration, liability, reimbursement/pay, and working conditions fall under the responsibility of the country where the nurse is employed or the country where she is actually practicing, that is, where the patient is? Problems have occurred when domestic banks outsource their services and contract for offshore financial analysis. What happens when the care of the sick is internationally outsourced?

In the United States, where professional regulation falls under the responsibility of each state, the challenge of interstate practice is currently being addressed. The National Council of State Boards of Nursing (NCSBN) supported the development of an Interstate Compact whose final text was adopted in 1997. Individual states may "elect to enact the Compact permitting nurses licensed in one state to practice in other states that also have enacted the Compact. Nurses are expected to abide by the laws of the state in which they are providing the service, i.e. the place where the client is to be found. . . . The model anticipates that the nurse will be licensed in the state of residence, rather than the state where the client is located—a radical departure from current practice."[21] This may serve as a model for international cross-border services.

Mode 2 covers what GATS calls *consumption abroad*. This involves a service supplied in the territory of one WTO member to the service consumer of any other WTO member. Consumption abroad includes the provision of education to foreign students, a very lucrative business already discussed in chapter 3. If patients, or in economic language "consumers," travel from one country to another to obtain a diagnosis or treatment from health systems considered better equipped, more specialized, cheaper, or of higher quality, they also fall under GATS mode 2. A good example is the Clinique de Genolier in Switzerland. The Clinique is located near both Geneva and Lausanne and boasts of its spectacular Alpine views, "wide therapeutic panorama," and "VIP services." It achieved world renown in the 1970s by offering specialized services, notably cardiovascular surgery, not only to Swiss patients but to groups of foreign patients, mostly from the former Yugoslavia and the Netherlands. These patients were prepared for surgery in their home countries, brought to the clinic for their surgical intervention, and returned home for rehabilitation once their stitches were removed.

The absence or insufficient quantity of specialized care in patients' home countries means that many either cannot get or must delay surgery. Patients in less-developed countries are not the only ones attracted to this commercial option. American patients are encouraged to go to Montreal to get vision correction surgery, which is less expensive there than in the United States. With the extra savings and thanks to a cheaper Canadian dollar, they can afford a pleasant holiday in the city. On the web, UK patients are informed that they can avoid long waits for cataract or glaucoma surgery at home if they hop on the boat train and check into a clinic in Calais, France.[22] Because so many patients are now lured by these obvious attractions, governments and private entrepreneurs are promoting trade negotiations that facilitate the newly coined "health tourism."

In some cases, public and private health insurance companies or systems cover the patients' expenses and finance the travel and living expenses of family members as well. When surgery or other services are more easily available abroad, even with the extra charges for family members, government-financed health systems and private insurers may find them to be quite cost-effective. The Canadian government health system, for example, often sends cancer patients from Toronto or Montreal to get their chemotherapy in Buffalo, New York, or in Burlington, Vermont, because it is cheaper for the government to make use of American capacity than to spend the money on providing services at home. Similarly, the Samoan health system regularly refers patients to Australia and New Zealand, finding it more cost-effective to pay for certain procedures in a foreign country than maintain sophisticated equipment and highly specialized personnel locally.

This is a clear extension of traditional practices of patients crossing provincial or state boundaries within a given country to get treatment in regional or national centers specializing in a certain type of care not available locally. The interface between specialization and migration highlights an interesting dimension of the migration process.

Several developing countries have found their market niche in offering a specific type of care or combining health services with tourism and recreational packages. Jintana Yunibhand, president of the Thai Nurses Association, explains that health tourism is expanding rapidly along the coastal areas in Thailand and offers attractive employment as well as entrepreneurial opportunities for nurses. On the web, Thai health facilities and tourism agencies offer "executive medical tourism" packages. Announcements claim, for example, that the savings on one "major tooth repair" can pay for an economy-rate two-week vacation. They go on to target the many US residents without health insurance. Since all aspects of American health care are overpriced, they argue, health tourism is an ideal choice for those without health care insurance.[23]

According to the Cuba Tourism Office, "along with those who seek the sun, white sands and warm waters, there are those interested in combining their vacations with a program that provides them with an ideal physical state, with the final goal of achieving a better quality of life."[24] Tom Fawthrop of BBC News agrees that the successful export of its medical technology abroad and health tourism within the country have boosted Cuba's struggling economy and improved the quality of life of its own population. In 2003 alone "more than 5000 foreign patients traveled to Cuba for a wide range of treatments including eye-surgery, neurological disorders such as multiple sclerosis and Parkinson's disease, and orthopaedics. The unique

Cuban treatment for retinitis pigmentosa, often known as night blindness, has attracted many patients from Europe and North America. . . . Health tourism generates revenues of around $40 million a year."[25] Nurses are obviously involved in all these treatments and care programs.

The third mode of trade in health services, called *commercial presence,* involves the flow of capital from one WTO member to another for the purpose of establishing a business. When, for example, an American company wants to establish a chain of hospitals in other countries, or a business in France wants to set up a diagnostic center in Morocco, then it moves into mode 3. Commercial presence facilitates a wide range of businesses—health care facilities, management consulting firms, labor recruitment agencies, information technology firms, and training facilities, to name only a few.

Rupa Chanda explains that "such ventures typically involve acquisition of facilities, management contracts, and licensing arrangements with some degree of local participation to ensure access to certified and adequately trained local persons and to ensure local contacts and commitment." He cites the example of the Singapore-based Parkway Group that "has acquired hospitals in Asia and Britain and has created an international chain of hospitals, Gleneagles International, through joint ventures with partners in Malaysia, Indonesia, Sri Lanka, India, and the UK. It has also set up a dental surgery chain through joint ventures in South-East Asia. . . . There are also emerging opportunities for firms with experience in accreditation, legislation, and medical standards."[26]

Local job creation is just one of the possible outcomes from private foreign investment of this type. In countries where there is unemployment or underemployment of the personnel required to provide the new services, job creation is likely to be a positive and welcome development. There is always the risk, however, that these new jobs may result in internal migration and deplete an already stretched labor market accessible to vital public services.[27] For example, the establishment of a private spa or cardio fitness center in a relatively deserted rural or coastal area may lure nurses away from working in the public service sector caring for the local population with access only to publicly funded free services. Depending on the pay and working conditions offered to the nurse, such a move may yield a significant improvement in her standard of living. For the local population, it might well mean a deterioration of the available health care.

Although various ethical codes attempt to control international migration, no such barriers or instruments exist to constrain internal flows of personnel from depleted public services to for-profit, private-sector employment. The internal movement of personnel may prove to be just as great and have very similar consequences, however.

While the kind of trade flows targeted in mode 3 tend to be from industrialized to developing countries, investment capital has been exchanged between developing countries. For example, the Apollo group of hospitals in India has begun constructing hospitals abroad and plans to invest a further $4 million to build fifteen new hospitals in Malaysia, Nepal, and Sri Lanka.[28] The overseas expansion of the South African enterprise Netcare is an example of a chain based in a developing country that is creating business opportunities in industrialized as well as other developing countries.

Finally, there is GATS mode 4—the *presence of natural persons* of a WTO member in the territory of any other WTO member. This comes into play when foreigners in a given country deliver health services. It is the counterpart of a "commercial presence" (mode 3)—the famous trade-off mentioned above between industrialized and developing countries. Since WTO decisions are made by consensus (agreement by all member states), incorporating the movement of labor into a section like mode 4 was essential if GATS was to be adopted. With regard to international nurse migration, GATS mode 4 is the most relevant.

In general, "the movement of a person from one country to another for economic reasons has at least three dimensions: length of stay, level of skills, and nature of the contract. Each dimension allows for significant variation."[29] The complexity of mode 4 becomes apparent as soon as countries enter into discussions. That is when this new creation—"the natural person"—moves to center stage and becomes the focus of different interpretations that tend to lead to heated debates.

How do these discussions and ambiguities affect nurse migration? Are they really significant? Discussions on GATS tend to take two directly opposite directions. Some health-sector stakeholders are convinced that mode 4 is taking over the world, while others feel just as strongly that it is irrelevant. Technically, mode 4 is defined in article 1.2(d) of GATS as being "the supply of a service . . . by a service supplier of one Member, through presence of natural persons of a Member in the territory of another Member."[30] An annex to GATS aims to clarify and provide greater detail on the characteristics of mode 4. It specifies that the agreement *does not* apply to natural persons seeking access to the employment market of another member country or to measures regarding citizenship, residence, or employment on a permanent basis. The annex goes on to say that mode 4 *does* refer to "natural persons who are service suppliers of a Member, and natural persons of a Member who are employed by a service supplier of a Member, in respect of the supply of a service."[31]

One would hope that reading this explanation would make the situation relatively clear. So after reviewing the text, Nurse Dupont[†] from France, who wishes to work in Vietnam for one year, should be able to understand whether she fits category mode 4 under GATS and has a good chance of getting a work permit. But no, the ambiguities are such that the situation is not clear at all. The critical inconsistency is the phrase "seeking access to the employment market." It seems contradictory to have natural persons working in a country and yet not integrate that country's employment market. How is this possible?

Many confess difficulty in understanding and sigh in despair. Indeed, rather than clarify, these additional definitions and qualifying exclusions lead to a great deal of confusion and a certain degree of legal uncertainty. Of the two categories presented in the annex and cited above, the first is quite straightforward. It refers to self-employed or independent service suppliers who obtain their remuneration directly from customers (individuals or enterprises)—for example, an Australian nurse practitioner who establishes a practice and offers direct services to chronically ill patients in Fiji, or a nurse management consultant from Sweden who opens a firm in Poland and advises a local hospital on its human resources management plan. The second—natural persons of a member country who are employed by a service supplier of a member—is not clear at all.

In addition to independent service providers, it is generally assumed that GATS mode 4 covers real people employed by a foreign service supplier. Mode 4 goes into action when that foreign service supplier obtains a contract to provide services and sends its employees to work in the host country company where they deliver the contracted services on a temporary basis. For example, the National Health Service in the United Kingdom contracts with Netcare of South Africa. Netcare sends its team of health care professionals to perform cataract surgery in London facilities for a period of three to six months. Mode 4 also governs a second type of employee status—foreigners who are employed abroad by foreign companies established in the host country—for example, a US-owned hospital/spa facility established in Thailand employing nurses from California on a temporary contract.

What remains ambiguous is whether or not GATS also covers instances where foreigners are employed by host country companies. Does GATS apply to a Filipino nurse working in Birmingham for the National Health Service of England? The annex specifically excludes the migrant worker seeking access to the employment market. This would suggest that the Filipino nurse would be exempt from GATS rules. Some governments disagree and insist the treaty applies. There has been no definitive decision with regard to this type of case under GATS. Yet, these are precisely the conditions that are the most relevant and apply to the great majority of migrant workers, including nurses.

If the ambiguity is not removed at the highest level, this matter will be one more condition negotiated bilaterally by WTO members when specific country commitments under the GATS framework are determined. In other words, under the GATS umbrella there may be a multitude of country-specific basic conditions and terminology creating a "spaghetti bowl" effect. This may allow flexibility but will necessarily result in a complex web of international legal instruments to monitor and apply, which will in all likelihood sow even more confusion.

The annex states that GATS will not apply to natural persons seeking permanent employment, therefore implying that it will only cover temporary workers. The problem is that when you search the document, you find it does not define the word *temporary*. Commentators have pointed out that "given that temporary entry under GATS commitments can last for up to 3 years (or in some cases longer), the service provider has in effect entered the local labor market, even though they are not applying for citizenship."[32] Again, the confusion and different interpretations are less than helpful when trying to understand GATS or to predict its future relevance and impact on individuals, services, and nations.

While mode 4 makes no differentiation between service suppliers with regard to skill level, in practice the benefits have generally gone to the higher-skilled or professionals: managers, executives, and specialists. Within this group intracompany transferees have predominated. These are staff members employed by a transnational corporation (a business with branches in more than one country) and transferred between the headquarters and a branch or between branches of the same enterprise. For example, a nurse employed by the Hospital Corporation of America, a transnational chain, could temporarily be transferred from the United States to provide short-term management consulting services in one of their hospitals in Switzerland. The industrialized countries support the present bias in favor of higher-skilled persons, whereas the developing countries, in an attempt to address unemployment issues at home, hope to broaden the commitments to include lower-skilled workers. Economists estimate that if the industrialized countries' temporary work quotas were increased by an amount equal to 3 percent of their current workforce, there would be an increase in world welfare of $156 billion per year.[33]

GATS leaves much to the interpretation of its members, and follow-up discussions are often frustrating, as representatives speak on a given issue using the same words but meaning different things. Part of the problem, as Rudolph Adlung and Antonia Carzaniga state, may be the "absence of well-established coordination between competent sectoral ministries and agencies on the one hand and the trade negotiators in charge of GATS on the other."[34]

Very little data are available, but recent estimates suggest that mode 1 (services supplied in one country to clients in another) and mode 3 (the transnational expansion of companies) each accounted for about two-fifths of the world trade in services. Mode 2 (the consumption of services abroad) contributed one-fifth, while trade considered under mode 4 (presence of natural persons as workers abroad) was found to be relatively insignificant.[35] GATS may facilitate nurse migration in the future, but only if "temporary" contracts extend to five years and if host companies are allowed to employ them. If this is not the case, only independent practitioners (estimated to be 1 percent of current nurses), an equally small minority of intracompany transferees, and nurses in their home countries with access to the new jobs created by foreign investment will be offered additional advantages under GATS. In spite of this verdict, GATS, in all its modes, still has a considerable effect on nurses, whether migrant or domestic.

Potential Opportunities and Threats

Ever since the first GATS talks there has been a great deal of discussion about its potential repercussions. The European Commission in 1999 came to the conclusion that "the GATS is not just something that exists between Governments. It is first and foremost an instrument for the benefit of business."[36] Critics of globalization from civil society—the general public, nonprofit private sector, and nongovernmental organizations—express legitimate concern that business interests will distort or threaten future accessibility to public services. Intergovernmental specialized agencies such as the WHO and the ILO share similar concerns. The failure of the ministerial conference in Cancun in September 2003 has delayed negotiations on GATS, and it is difficult to predict its future. In February 2004 Rubens Ricupero, secretary-general of the United Nations Conference on Trade and Development (UNCTAD), argued that "this is a round that nobody wants. But it has become politically incorrect to suggest that continuous trade negotiations are not necessary."[37]

Supporters of GATS claim that it promises economic development, which will lead to higher standards of living for the world's population. Increasing the markets for goods and services has the potential to create employment and entrepreneurial opportunities and to stimulate a more cost-effective use of resources. Expanded markets promise the delivery of a wider range of goods and services available for purchase or contract. They insist that greater access to accredited education and training would be facilitated, and eventually internationally recognized standards of quality and competence—the right to practice a profession—might develop.

Detractors of GATS claim just the opposite. A huge global movement of critics now includes such renowned figures as Joseph Stiglitz, who won the Nobel Prize for economics in 2001 and was chief economist for the World Bank between 1997 and 2000. Stiglitz talks about the backlash against globalization. In *Globalization and Its Discontents* he writes that "few—apart from those with vested interests who benefit from keeping out the goods produced by the poor countries—defend the hypocrisy of pretending to help developing countries by forcing them to open up their markets to the goods of the advanced industrial countries while keeping their own markets protected, policies that make the rich richer and the poor more impoverished— and increasingly angry."[38]

Other critics document that globalization has heightened unequal distribution of increased wealth nationally and internationally. "Economic globalization has resulted in divergence between economies—faster growth in the richest and slower growth in the poorest—and has been blamed for increasing inequality within countries and slower poverty reduction in low-income countries. . . . The contribution of growth to poverty reduction depends critically on the distribution of the associated increase in incomes."[39] Trade may indeed support inequality both internationally and domestically unless corrective measures and safeguards are put in place.

There is an obvious and inherent push within GATS to promote the privatization of services, which will then compete with or replace the public sector. This will potentially limit access for poor populations and create a two-tiered system based on the consumer's ability to pay. Increased private or commercial influence on national and international policies threatens public accountability and universal access to basic services such as health, education, and even water. Dominant corporate interests could determine and define the public good. The health sector has been spared from aggressive GATS negotiations in many countries. Jealously guarded as a public service, it has so far been purposefully excluded from GATS by most countries. There is cause to be vigilant, however, as the integrity of public services, especially fringe services, is under attack nationally and soon will be internationally. For example, the extended privatization of insurance (including health insurance) may distort eligibility and coverage criteria, leading to greater inequities in the delivery of services among segments of the population.[40] In health care, for example, community risk-sharing is replaced by admitting only low-health-risk individuals (and therefore less costly clients) as policyholders.

At the same time, the complete absence of any reference to core labor standards in GATS may threaten workers' rights to a decent wage, a safe work environment, and freedom of association. It is ironic that the largest traders in the world—the United States and the European Union—advocate linking labor and environmental standards with trade. The opposition comes foremost from developing countries—Indonesia, India, Brazil—which have come to believe from past experience that industrialized countries will use these labor and environment standards as a means of increasing production costs abroad and thereby "protect" their sectors from competition from developing countries.

The conflicting vested interests in globalization have produced a flurry of monitoring groups that track the impact of trade negotiations. One of them is GATSwatch, a joint project of the Corporate Europe Observatory and the Transnational Institute, which provides research and analysis of the role and agenda of corporate lobbies with regard to GATS negotiations. On the home page of its website, the group readily acknowledges that it supports global networking against GATS.[41] According to GATSwatch, the complete absence of a comprehensive assessment of the impact of GATS-style liberalization (the opening of national markets to international competition) is a significant concern. Recalling that the international trade in services is relatively new, they caution against negotiators forging ahead in unknown areas with no way to turn back if the chosen path proves to be detrimental to society as a whole. One thing is obvious—once health sectors are opened to foreign competition, they will never be the same.

Chanda points out that "many of the adverse implications of trade in health services . . . are due to internal factors, rather than to globalization per se. Moreover, while globalization may aggravate some of these problems, it may also provide opportunities for correcting some of the underlying conditions that are the root causes. . . . The impact of trade in health services for equity, access, costs, and quality of health services is largely dependent on the policies and safeguards governments put in place and on the existing conditions in the sector."[42] GATS detractors worry, however, that these safeguards will not be there when they are needed. The general confusion one experiences when reading the trade documents analyzed above underscores the legitimacy of this concern.

The growing public distrust of government is a phenomenon that commentators and researchers have noted worldwide. Nurses are part of this skeptical public. After all, many of them are very aware that government decisions in the 1980s led to the downsizing of the health sector, reduction of education placements, and substitution of qualified health personnel with lesser-trained staff—measures that helped create the present critical nursing shortage. They no longer trust governments to protect either them or their patients. The basic question therefore is: Will governments introduce or maintain the safeguards necessary to ensure equitable access to basic services, or will they promote economic development for some at the expense of others?

When nurses become aware of the power of trade agreements, one of their biggest worries is that GATS has the potential to weaken, restrict, or replace government and professional regulatory mechanisms and structures that ensure quality services. One critical example would be the assessment of professional qualifications of foreign nurses. Under pressure from trade negotiators, and possibly from ministries of foreign affairs, there are attempts to standardize or harmonize nurses' qualifications so that the meaning of the term *registered nurse* is the same in every country. This effort would create a standardized education, a one-size-fits-all nursing curriculum that would be offered worldwide. The harmonization of qualification standards could raise educational standards. However, it is more likely to lead to competency levels being lowered to meet the minimum standards of the widest possible range of countries. Many nurses and nursing groups argue that a four-year university education for entry into practice will produce nurses who can better deal with the complexities of modern health care and provide better care to patients. Nurses and patients will suffer, they insist, if the priority of global health care businesses is to manufacture nurses for export as quickly and cheaply as possible. There is already evidence that market forces are eroding the regulations and restrictions that governments and private professional associations create and impose.[43] Patient safety and service improvements could be seriously threatened by such trends.

The World Trade Organization

In the light of massive demonstrations and widespread protests, the World Trade Organization secretariat has attempted to provide reassurance and clarification on GATS and its related processes. A fact sheet available on the WTO website titled "Misunderstandings and Scare Stories" attempts to respond to common concerns.[44] It insists that governments are free to choose those services on which they will make commitments guaranteeing access to foreign suppliers. The WTO points out that many public services (like health and education) are not provided on a commercial or competitive basis and therefore not subject to GATS. The WTO secretariat repeatedly attempts to remind the public that GATS focuses on trade and purposely distances itself from immigration policy, labor standards, and development issues. The WTO says it claims no mandate in these areas. There is inevitably a link, however, and the resistance to deal with these issues generates a great deal of frustration, distrust, and ill will. Needless to say, this stance adds to the confusion that surrounds discussions about the meaning and application of global trade agreements.

Here is one of the main problem areas. The WTO claims that the right of governments to regulate is one of the fundamental premises of GATS. The organization insists that the objective of GATS is to liberalize services trade and not deregulate services. In other words, professions that have strict criteria for entry into practice, like physicians and nurses, will continue to set standards nationally (or by state/province). This makes a distinction between a work permit (the right to employment) and a license (the right to practice). For example, Nurse Marshall[†] from Jamaica may obtain the right to work in the United States, but unless she passes the NCLEX-RN licensing exam, she will not be able to work as a nurse.

The WTO fact sheet emphasizes that the organization does not set international standards nor does it review national standards. It is only interested in qualification requirements and procedures, technical standards, and licensing requirements if they have the potential to constitute unnecessary barriers to trade in services.

Disciplines and Professional Regulation

This narrowly focused review of professional regulation ("domestic regulation" in GATS) is introduced in article 6 of GATS, which mandates the Council for Trade in Services to develop what it calls *disciplines*. The accounting profession was chosen as a priority because the profession had already taken significant steps to internationalize standards and because accounting services are critical to international trade.[45] In December 1998 the WTO's Council for Trade in Services adopted the Disciplines on Domestic Regulation in the Accountancy Sector. They address objectives, transparency, prior notice and consultation, licensing requirements and procedures, equivalency issues, and technical standards. According to a WTO press release, "Most professional services . . . are heavily regulated, and for good reasons: but it is also true that regulations can be an unnecessary, and usually unintended, barrier to trade in services."[46] The Accountancy Disciplines were developed as a model. There is now a working party to see if they can be generalized to other professions so as to avoid drafting endless profession-specific texts, which would be too time-consuming and costly.

Many professional associations and regulatory bodies viewed this development with concern. Nursing groups quickly realized that trade considerations had the potential to compromise their mandate to advocate for and protect patients. They also recognized that these definitions and arrangements could present a serious danger to the professionals whose education and practice standards may be under attack. In an attempt to respond to these concerns, article 3 of the Accountancy Disciplines allows for the protection of consumers, quality assurance of services, professional competence of service providers (adequate skill levels), and assurance of professional integrity. This text may be easily adapted to pertain to health instead of accountancy.

> Members shall ensure that measures . . . relating to licensing requirements and procedures, technical standards and qualification requirements and procedures are not prepared, adopted or applied with a view to or with the effect of creating unnecessary barriers to trade in accountancy services. For this purpose, Members shall ensure that such measures are not more trade-restrictive than necessary to fulfil a legitimate objective. Legitimate objectives are, *inter alia*, the protection of consumers (which includes all users of accounting services and the public generally), the quality of the service, professional competence, and the integrity of the profession.[47]

Needless to say, professional regulation (and in the new GATS terminology, disciplines) has a direct impact on international migration of nurses. It is the key that will open the door to employment with the right to practice as a professional in another country. While GATS is not directly involved in setting standards, member governments can be challenged to demonstrate that a given measure is not more trade-restrictive than necessary. The costly legal and bureaucratic process that may follow such a challenge may influence the final outcome of a negotiated dispute judgment, possibly to the detriment of professional standards. Take a country like Australia, which now has a bachelor's degree as the minimal level of education in order to practice as a nurse. It may be challenged to prove that this is really necessary and not just a protective measure to prevent nurses from other countries without a university degree from getting employment in Australia. The legal battles may be very lengthy and expensive. The risk is that the high standards of nursing education in Australia will be compromised and lowered to meet trade considerations.

Bilateral, Multilateral, and Regional Trade Agreements

While GATS attracts a great deal of attention and has become the standard against which other trade agreements are compared, many others are already in effect or being developed. Although their signatories, scope, and purpose may differ, every one of them may influence international nurse migration. Generally, agreements among countries enjoying geographic proximity, close cultural and historical ties, and similar levels of development take a more liberal approach to labor mobility than agreements among geographically distant members with differing levels of development.[48]

Some regional trade agreements cover the mobility of people in general (including permanent migrants and nonworkers); others offer free movement of workers (including entry to the local labor market); some are restricted to facilitating the movement of certain kinds of trade- or investment-related activities; and yet others are limited to addressing a specific category of movement, for example, temporary workers or, as with GATS, service suppliers. In most cases, governments retain broad discretion to grant, refuse, and administer residence permits and visas.[49]

Julia Nielson, now with the World Bank, has developed a very helpful classification of regional trade agreements which analyzes their approach to labor mobility. This is of importance to any discussion of nurse migration.[50] Nielson explains that agreements providing market access for certain groups include the Caribbean Community (CARICOM). Its Protocol II on Establishment, Services, and Capital (1998) provides free movement of university graduates, other professionals and skilled persons, and selected occupations as well as freedom of travel and exercise of a profession.[51] From a nursing perspective what is interesting is that a mutual recognition agreement between countries of this region existed previously to the protocol. Since 1993, after a harmonization of the nursing curricula, nurses in over ten Caribbean countries began taking a common licensure exam. This led to the mutual recognition of credentials and almost complete regional mobility.[52] In other words, Nurse Clarke from Barbados has complete freedom to emigrate to Jamaica or Belize or Saint Lucia and start practicing as a nurse—without taking any further exams or any special supervised programs.

Other well-known examples of this type of regional trade agreement are the North American Free Trade Agreement (NAFTA) between Canada, Mexico and the United States, and chapter K of the Canada-Chile Free Trade Agreement. The measures presented in these documents are limited to temporary entry and facilitate the movement of traders and investors, intracompany transferees, business visitors (usually very short term stays), and professionals, although visas and professional accreditation are still required. Regulatory bodies retain significant freedom to develop unilateral or bilateral approaches to the recognition of another country's licensing criteria. Regulation in Canada and the United States falls under the responsibility of the provinces and states. Standards, procedures, and criteria vary from jurisdiction to jurisdiction and from profession to profession. Canada, under the Agreement on Internal Trade, is committed to remove or reduce interprovincial barriers to the movement of workers, goods, services, and capital.[53] While mutual recognition agreements may be difficult internationally, federated countries may have the same challenges internally. This will affect internal mobility as well as international migration. Nurse Baker with a nursing degree from Manitoba may need to be screened as a "foreign" nurse if he wants to work in Québec or Ontario, thus prolonging the internal migration process.

Some trade agreements have modified the GATS model. The US-Jordan Free Trade Agreement, for example, adds specific visa commitments, and its scope goes beyond service suppliers. The EU-Mexico Free Trade Agreement, although not yet in effect, goes beyond GATS by introducing regulation of work, labor conditions, and permanent residency of natural persons. Other agreements, such as the Southern Common Market Agreement (MERCO-SUR), replicate the GATS model exactly.

After beginning as an informal dialogue group, the Asia Pacific Economic Cooperation (APEC) Forum has become the primary regional vehicle for promoting open trade and practical economic cooperation. This group of countries now represents an impressive 45 percent of global trade. APEC does not address market access but facilitates labor mobility for intracompany transfers and specialists while ignoring the self-employed and unskilled or semiskilled workers. The creation of an APEC Business Travel Card facilitates the entry of business visitors. Valid for three years, it provides multiple short-term business entries, with stays of two or three months on each arrival. At present, this agreement has benefited traditional commercial and business enterprises, especially transnational companies that transfer their staff for short periods or send consultants to work on specific projects. As the private health industry develops, these conditions may also apply to health professionals, including nurses—keeping in mind that professional accreditation will still be an issue.

Another set of agreements, the Central European Free Trade Agreement (CEFTA), focuses exclusively on trade and does not contain provisions on labor mobility or services. This agreement, adopted in 1991, created a free trade area and proclaimed a declaration of cooperation between Poland, Czech Republic, Slovakia, Hungary, Slovenia, Romania, and Bulgaria. CEFTA is said to function as a preparation for full EU membership, and relations among member countries are founded on the principles of the market economy.

Finally, some regional trade agreements provide full mobility of labor. One example is the Trans-Tasman Travel Arrangement, a follow-up of the Services Protocol of the Australia–New Zealand Closer Economic Relations Agreement. Australians and New Zealanders are free to live and work anywhere in these two countries for indefinite periods of time. As with the CARICOM countries, a mutual recognition agreement exists. In other words, a registered nurse from New Zealand will automatically have the right to practice in Australia.

Another good example of this type of regional trade agreement is the European Community Treaty negotiated by the European Union, where full mobility is considered one of the four fundamental freedoms of the single market. In principle, the treaty guarantees its citizens the right to move and reside freely within any of the member states (recently expanded from fifteen to twenty-five in May 2004) as well as the freedom of movement of workers, the right of establishment for the self-employed, and the freedom to provide services.

European Nursing Directives

In the early years when it was called the European Economic Community,[54] "much effort and many resources were devoted to the development of 'sectoral directives' that regulated the movement of licensed professionals across the borders of the member states so that the Treaty's provision for free movement of labor could apply to them along with unregulated workers. Nursing was among the sectors dealt with by the Commission."[55] In 1977 the Council of Ministers approved the EC Nursing Sectoral Directives, which became effective in 1979. They provide for the mutual recognition of diplomas awarded in all fifteen nations in membership at the time. In principle, therefore, a nurse with a diploma from an EU nation, for example, Portugal, Italy, Germany, Holland, the United Kingdom, or France, is allowed to practice nursing in any of the EU member states. No work permit is required.

A status report released in 1994 by the Advisory Committee on Training in Nursing suggested there was considerable divergence in the actual practices of the member states and that automatic recognition was not being applied in all cases. These apparent breaches of the agreement demonstrate the sometimes difficult task of international credentialing or recognition of qualifications when a common exam is not an integral part of the process. For example, if a national regulatory body from one country, say, the United Kingdom, felt that the curriculum in community nursing in another country, perhaps Holland or Italy, was not comprehensive enough, it would refuse to recognize the Dutch or Italian nurse's diploma and demand a supervised adaptation period, as would be the case for many other foreign nurses from countries outside the European Union. While this would be in breach of the EU agreement, the practice has been formally challenged in only rare cases.

In principle, a nurse whose foreign qualifications have been recognized by one EU country should be able to practice nursing in any other EU member state (the issue of work permits put aside). For example, a South African–educated nurse now registered in the United Kingdom may assume she has the right to practice in Germany, France, or Belgium. The automatic third-country recognition has, however, been challenged through the EU Commission, and the rules still need to be clarified if they are to be applied consistently.

Within the European Union there was concern that sectoral directives were too expensive to develop and maintain. Similarities with the streamlined approach used with regard to the GATS disciplines are obvious—going from a profession-specific to a more widely applicable text. The push for generic language led to the adoption of the General Systems Directive, which determined that all persons recognized as a professional in one EU member state must be recognized as such in another member state. This directive could have had a significant impact on nurses in the ten accession countries that recently became members. If their nurses fell under the General Systems Directive, they would automatically be registered throughout the European Union. In fact, nurses continue to fall under the specific responsibility of the 1977 Nursing Sectoral Directives.

Extensive country visits by an expert "peer review" group, appointed and funded by the European Commission, were undertaken to evaluate the education programs in each of the accession countries. The expert teams concluded that the level of nursing education, although improving, was not yet at the level demanded by the 1997 directives. Once the commission released the results of these reviews, nursing associations of the traditional EU countries did a great deal of lobbying to make sure that the professional recognition of these nurses continues to be under the responsibility of the Nursing Sectoral Directives. This would impose in many cases a significant upgrading of the current nursing education as a precondition to practice in another EU country. Equally necessary would be bridging courses for nurses having already graduated—education programs targeting the gaps in nurses' knowledge and skills so that they are able to meet the current and higher EU practice standards. As with nurses from countries outside the European Union, their qualifications and diplomas are carefully screened, and the need for adaptation periods is determined on a case-by-case basis.

The review of nursing education in Poland is a case in point. The European Commission report highlighted serious deficiencies in that former Eastern bloc country, namely, inadequate length and content of nursing education programs and insufficient evidence that changes are being implemented at a reasonable pace.[56] Despite this negative report, the European Union at its Copenhagen Summit of December 2002 granted Polish nurses the automatic right to practice in any of the member states. The Nursing and Midwifery Council and the Royal College of Nursing in the United Kingdom wrote a joint letter to their foreign secretary to voice their grave concerns about the "lack of sufficient nurse-led nursing education institutions, length of training for basic registration and the inappropriate division of hours of study between theory and practice."[57] They stressed that most nurses trained in Poland have to undergo an adaptation program of at least six months before they join the UK register, a clear indication of the discrepancies in the existing education. Similar letters from a variety of sources were sent to the European Commission and the minister of health in Poland. The president of the Polish Nurses Association joined the president of the Standing Committee of Nurses in the European Union in writing a cosigned letter to the European commissioner and relevant Polish ministers. Rather than upholding the decision for what was considered to be ill-advised automatic professional recognition, they urged the establishment of appropriate education upgrading programs in Poland. Clearly the Polish nurses themselves saw this as a welcome opportunity and pressure to upgrade the nursing education and advance the profession in their country.

This response underlines the complexity of the issue. While some see professional registration as an unnecessary barrier to the mobility of personnel, Adam Smith, the father of market theory, long ago understood that regulation can actually support the expansion of markets. It does so by assuring customers, or in this case patients, that the services provided by professionals will not jeopardize their health. Ultimately, the people who suffer the most from the absence of a credible professional assessment system are patients who unknowingly entrust their care to nurses whose qualifications are either false or do not meet local standards. Automatic recognition in this case discourages other accession countries from dutifully upgrading their education programs to meet higher standards and removes the incentive to improve or advance the profession. At the end of 2003 David Amos, deputy human resources director at the Department of Health (England), was "still unclear about whether the qualifications and work experience of those wishing to move to the UK from these states (accession countries) would be recognized automatically."[58] Decisions taken in mid-2004, however, did uphold the Nursing Sectoral Directives. In order to safeguard the agreed-upon education standards and protect the public, the EU affirmed the authority of national regulatory bodies within the traditional EU member countries to screen nurses with diplomas from the ten accession countries.

Another troubling regulatory shortcut or bypass on the trade superhighway was attempted by the European Union. In the autumn of 2002, the strong drive to recruit nurses to the industrialized countries produced a proposal that European nurses (with a minimum of two years' experience) be allowed to practice unregistered for sixteen weeks in the country of their choice. Not only nursing associations and the regulatory bodies but the Consumers' Association strongly opposed this initiative. The Consumers' Association declared that this proposal could "create a market where poorly qualified or dangerous professionals are imported and exported throughout the EU."[59] A coalition of parties opposed to the EU proposal argued that professionals who had been struck off the register in one country could be allowed to practice in another if registration screening procedures were ignored. This would mean that Nurse Nolan[†], struck off the register in Ireland for abusing a patient, could with impunity find work as a nurse in the United Kingdom for four months. Nothing would prevent Nolan from then going to work for another period of four months in a different EU member country, and the carousel ride continues.

In December 2003 the European Parliament's legal affairs committee amended the proposed legislation, and members agreed that all health professionals must register in the country where they provide services, no matter how briefly they plan to stay.[60] It will be interesting to see how the United Kingdom accommodates the previously mentioned South African nurses employed by Netcare and working for short durations in Britain.

The problems here are legion. Nurses who have the right to move to another country but do not meet the professional registration criteria always run the risk of being hired as auxiliaries and exploited by unscrupulous employers. Alternative and more constructive approaches are often sadly missing. The solution would be to upgrade preregistration nursing education in the source countries. Another possibility is to offer bridge or conversion courses—shorter programs that focus on making up the differences between the nursing education of different countries, for example, between Poland and the United Kingdom, or China and the United States. These measures would be most cost-effective if nurses were provided easy access to them in terms of location, scheduling, and expenses.

Mutual Recognition Agreements

The establishment of legally enforced, internationally accepted education standards is one way to ensure a common level of service provision while having the advantage of enabling greater mobility of professionals. In recent years the Philippine Nurses Association has repeatedly pushed for the development of global nursing education norms that would facilitate registration procedures for its migrant nurses. The different levels of nursing education worldwide reflect the global variations in the legal status of nurses and the scope of their activities. In fact, there is no consensus that it is even feasible or desirable to have globally recognized nursing education standards. Even at the national level, the recognition and utilization of skills are sometimes determined by local cultures or resources. The nurse in an isolated rural community might provide services that in well-staffed urban centers are exclusively given by physicians. Some groups, including the World Health Organization, have argued that national norms and standards are essential to respond both to country-specific circumstances and health needs. Many nurses fear that high global standards are not feasible at this time and attempts to harmonize the norms will harm the profession by debasing the quality of education to the lowest common denominator.

Because of these heated debates, national regulatory bodies like the Canadian Nurses Association and international organizations like the International Council of Nurses (ICN) feel that it is more productive to avoid a focus on rigid qualification assessments (diplomas, degrees, etc.) and instead determine the basic competencies (levels of performance demonstrating the effective application of knowledge, skill, and judgment) required to function as a qualified nurse. One example is the recently disseminated *Framework of Competencies for the Generalist Nurse.* "ICN, by virtue of its global leadership role in nursing, and the fact that it represents the voice of nursing internationally, considers that the time is right to establish international competencies for the generalist nurse," says Judith Oulton, ICN chief executive officer.[61] The ICN believes that these competencies will help clarify the role of nurses and guide future mutual recognition agreements and multicountry licensure programs. It urges countries to build upon the ICN framework while developing additional competencies that reflect the country-specific requirements of the nursing workforce.

The competencies for the generalist nurse, as set out by the ICN Framework, are grouped under three headings: (*a*) professional, ethical, and legal practice, (*b*) care provision and management, and (*c*) professional development. All competencies are given equal relevance and cover areas such as health promotion, assessment, and planning; implementation, evaluation, and accountability; therapeutic communication; safety; and delegation/supervision. Finally, professional enhancement, quality improvement, and continuing education are considered critical responsibilities of each and every practicing nurse.[62] Although it seems a long way off, identifying the core nurse competencies at the national level may pave the way for international standards. Such standards would present a clear picture of the role and duties of the nurse, reinforce patient safety mechanisms, provide a basis for curriculum development, and facilitate free movement of nurses globally.

The setting of national standards is the direct responsibility of either governments (usually ministries of health) or delegated authorities such as professional or self-regulatory bodies. The formal adoption of a common set of standards by the competent authorities of different countries is often the basis for negotiating mutual recognition agreements (MRAs).

These standards may be government-to-government agreements, but they are frequently managed and enforced by responsible professional bodies operating under delegated authority or independent from government. Some uncertainty is introduced when government-to-government agreements, such as GATS, must necessarily link with MRAs negotiated by independent professional groups. The recognition of qualifications is seen as a necessary corollary to market access under mode 4—which governs service providers who contract to work in a foreign country. Access to foreign employment will be severely limited if the qualifications of the service provider, in this case nurses, are not recognized by the destination country's regulatory body.[63]

"In terms of professional qualifications," Julia Nielson observes, "mutual recognition usually refers to both the recognition of the equivalence of the content of the training and to the recognition of the home country's authority to certify such training through the granting of diplomas or other evidence of qualification."[64] It is usually requested for academic purposes (to enroll in further education) or as a precondition for obtaining the right to exercise a licensed profession.

Although the services will be provided in the destination country, mutual recognition agreements essentially allocate regulatory jurisdiction to the source country. Consider the example of an Australian nurse who wants to work in a New Zealand health care center. In accordance with the Trans-Tasman Travel Arrangement, New Zealand authorizes and accepts the assessment of Australian-educated nurses made by a foreign entity, the regulatory body of Australia. If the Australian regulatory body decides that the nurse is qualified to practice in Australia, she will be granted permission and issued a license to practice in New Zealand.

Nielson explains that many so-called mutual recognition agreements "do not provide for automatic recognition of qualifications. Some are far-reaching (e.g., within the EU/EEA, or recognition of educational qualifications amongst the Baltic States), others provide for reduced requirements or procedures; some provide a degree of facilitation; others are limited to broader types of cooperation or dialogue."[65] Where there are differences in the scope of licensed activities between the countries, the agreement authorizes the destination country to impose additional requirements, or compensatory measures, for recognition. For example, nurses who are expected to give intravenous medications in the destination country but not in the source country may be required to successfully complete a special training course to acquire this skill before being fully registered to give such treatment in the destination country.

Mutual recognition is usually based on the principle of equivalence, providing countries a degree of flexibility in meeting any specific health needs of their populations. The professionals educated in countries that have signed a mutual recognition agreement tend therefore to have *equivalent* levels of skill (equal in value and content) or *comparable* qualifications (equal in value but not necessarily in content). For example, the hospital environment and access to equipment in the United Kingdom and in Italy may not be exactly the same. The range of practical nursing experience and clinical care provided will therefore be slightly different and yet contain all the essential elements to provide the necessary skill development in this particular area of care. In other words, the nurse trained in a medical/surgical ward in the United Kingdom may not have exactly the same clinical experience as the nurse in Italy, but it is considered comparable or equivalent.

Full harmonization of basic nursing education curricula and licensure has taken place within CARICOM, but this is a rare exception due to the difficulty in arriving at consensus and accommodating different national legal systems. "MRAs are easier to achieve when some harmonization of standards has already occurred," Pat Cutshall explains in her monograph on the regulation of cross-border professional regulation. "Bilateral agreements may be more easily reached than multilateral agreements and are likely to set the stage for the later addition of other parties to the agreement."[66]

Most MRAs tend to be established between developed countries that share a given region, culture, and history, like Australia and New Zealand or the Nordic countries. They rely on "common standards of training, common ethics and practices, and sometimes common cultures, languages and laws. MRAs are the optimal but also the most difficult type of arrangements to achieve."[67] Lack of progress made in this area may be attributed to the frequent absence of sophisticated regulatory bodies in developing countries.

For example, in many of the Francophone African countries, like Senegal, there is no systematic registration by an independent regulatory body. In addition, fear of losing national regulation sovereignty, and insufficient resources to devote to the frequently long and complex negotiations and follow-up monitoring, are significant obstacles which discourage attempts to make MRAs a widespread reality.

MRAs tend to be demand driven. The incentive to create an MRA almost always stems from an awareness that it will facilitate trade in services. For example, certain poorer countries in APEC are interested in exporting their nurses to wealthier APEC countries that are experiencing shortages. These countries have been inspired by the success of the Philippines. APEC members initiated exploratory discussions on the development of mutual recognition of nursing qualifications in 2003. Countries grappling with the burden of massive unemployment consider MRAs a good investment.

The limited number of MRAs implies that nurse migration is significantly restricted, but obviously this is not the case. The magnitude of migration flows in the past decades demonstrates that countries have processes in place to assess the qualifications of foreign-educated nurses. Where there are real trade interests, solutions are found.

Qualification Assessments

Where automatic recognition does not apply, the assessment of "paper qualifications"—diplomas or degrees received after the initial education program as opposed to current competencies or skills—is the most common form of professional recognition process. The review may be under the responsibility of a government agency or a professional regulatory body, for example, the Nursing and Midwifery Council of the United Kingdom.

According to Robyn Iredale from the University of Wollongong, Australia, "All of these bodies face similar problems of the cost of compiling and keeping their databases up-to-date, on deciding whether to assess institutions or individuals for comparability, 'substantial' equivalence or 'full' equivalence." Iredale adds, "They often reject qualifications that are not listed in their database due to the lack of knowledge or lack of precedents."[68] While unlisted qualifications are most likely to affect applicants from developing countries, they may influence decisions on nurses from unfamiliar industrialized countries as well. For example, Lesleyanne Hawthorne found that nurses from West Germany, Hong Kong, and Scandinavia had extremely low recognition rates in Australia—"not because of the inadequacy of their training, but due to lack of Australian research on the actual caliber of their courses."[69] This situation was corrected only after the regulatory body sent investigative teams to those countries to do an in-depth evaluation of their nursing education programs.

All of this is further complicated by barriers to the development of accurate tests of foreign nurses' knowledge as well as their clinical and language skills. In general, only nurses who have provided proof of registration in another country are eligible for an assessment, which may take the form of an exam or supervised clinical placement. The Australian Nursing Council has developed a test that is taken by domestic students before licensure as well as migrant nurses wishing to work in the country. It also provides preliminary and concurrent training for foreigners, which includes orientation to Australian nursing practice, the health system, culture, and medical terminology. In addition, the council presents a systematic overview of core nursing content—anatomy, physiology, pharmaceuticals, etc. The professional recognition success rate of foreign nurses has greatly improved since its introduction in the late 1980s.

Probationary working periods have been introduced as an assessment measure, usually in cases of critical shortages when staff is needed to take up work as soon as possible. Proof of registration in the home country and a minimum of work experience are normally required, and there has always been a strong resistance from professional bodies, and more recently from the consumers themselves, to even a temporary waiving of recognition screening because of the life-threatening risks involved. The attempted EU initiative allowing homegrown nurses to work in any of the member states for sixteen weeks before needing to register was rejected with these very same arguments.

Some of the measures used to test migrant nurses have been criticized in the past because of their expense and inherent bias. The cost of exams may be prohibitive for persons from developing countries, especially if travel to the destination country is required. Pretest and licensing exam centers are, however, being established in an increasing number of countries—yet more proof that encouraging nurse migration is considered good business and profitable trade.

Because tests often consist of multiple-choice questions, a format unfamiliar to many, migrant nurses are at an immediate disadvantage. Exams also tend to be culture specific. In order to respond accurately to the questions, knowledge of the destination country is necessary. To address this bias, foreign nurses—for example, Filipino and South Korean—have been hired in the United States to screen and suggest revisions of their pretest and licensing exams to ensure as much as possible culture-neutral wording and references in the exams.

While it is true that migrant nurses once employed in a foreign country will be dealing with patients that have a different cultural background, the purpose of these exams is to test professional and technical knowledge as well as analytical and problem-solving skills. To be objective, the process requires culture-neutral questions. This does not, however, negate the cultural differences between the migrant nurse and patient or the migrant nurse and colleagues. Rather, it emphasizes the need for comprehensive cultural orientation programs once the migrant nurse begins her employment contract.

Globalization is one of the most significant characteristics of this century. The push for economic growth and expanding markets has led to a focus on the international trade in services as well as the trade in goods. An interest in the global movement of capital has been accompanied by the demand for measures to support a greater movement in labor. Mode 4 of GATS has the potential to facilitate international nurse mobility if the questions of professional recognition and quality assurance of services are adequately addressed.

As mentioned, some trade negotiators consider the complex recognition process a protectionist measure on the part of the professions and an unnecessary barrier to trade and migration. An increasing number of groups including consumers, however, defend the accreditation process as a mechanism to ensure patient safety.

Mutual recognition agreements are complex, time consuming, and resource intensive. They demand a sophisticated infrastructure to ensure credible negotiations as well as informed decision making. MRAs are seen as the optimal and most effective method of recognition. Experts agree, however, that at present the variation in educational preparation, licensing systems, and national legal infrastructures is such that a truly global MRA will not become a reality for many years to come.

Other processes for the credentialing and professional recognition of foreign-educated professionals exist and continue to evolve. There is no doubt that the facilitated movement of licensed professionals depends on efficient recognition procedures. This begs the question, is more nurse migration really the desired goal? Part of the answer lies in an analysis and evaluation of the impact of international nurse migration on countries around the world.

6. Brain Drain, Brain Gain, Brain Circulation

Health systems all over the globe are faced with the challenge of recruiting qualified nurses and retaining them in active practice. Labor ministries are trying to maintain an efficient and effective workforce that responds positively to demographic changes in the population as well as to labor market forces. Finance ministries seek to encourage business interests that increase financial investment and economic growth. Humanitarian development agencies promote initiatives that support a worldwide campaign against poverty. Now, enter international nurse recruitment and migration—part of the solution for some of these, at times, conflicting imperatives or concerns, part of the problem for others.

As noted earlier, the international migration flow can be dramatic. Today, there are more Bangladeshi nurses in the Middle East than in Bangladesh.[1] In the 1970s already, there were more Filipino nurses registered in the United States and Canada than in the Philippines.[2] Even though this kind of migration is not a new phenomenon, its grand scale and directional shifts have never been seen before. Not surprisingly, as characteristics of international migration undergo change, new issues arise.

Africa and the Caribbean highlight many of the recent trends. Recently, the average annual number of Zimbabwean nurse registrations in the United Kingdom was higher than the number of nurses graduating in Zimbabwe in any given year, destroying any hope of workforce renewal or expansion in that southern African country.[3] Ghana's loss of 382 nurses through international migration in 1999 represented 100 percent of the annual output of its nursing schools.[4] Two-thirds of the Jamaican nurse graduates of the last twenty years are reported to have emigrated.[5] DENOSA (the nurses' professional union of South Africa) estimates that three hundred nurses leave the country every *month* to practice abroad, and in Zimbabwe the situation is even worse. The Community Working Group on Health estimates that two thousand nurses left that country each month in 2003.[6]

Then there is the Middle East and Asia. In the United Arab Emirates, foreigners accounted for nearly 98 percent of the 4,417 nurses employed in hospitals and other health facilities in 1999—a common profile for most of the Gulf States.[7] Enaam Abou Youssef (acting chief nursing scientist in the WHO) explains that the reliance on foreign nurses in these countries is unabated. "At times, an entire recruiting team from the Ministry of Health conducts the recruitment sessions, supported by their embassies established in the source countries. Both the private and public health sectors are recruiting foreign nurses."

In any given week, one nurse reports, seven thousand foreign nurse interviews are held by Saudi health employers and their representatives. It is not surprising that in 1999 the WHO found 84 percent of the nurses employed in Saudi Arabia to be expatriates, while only 16 percent were nationals. Depending on their countries of origin, nurses were paid different salaries. Recruits from the United States, the United Kingdom, and Australia were given preferential treatment and tended to receive higher salaries than those from developing countries (Philippines, China, Bangladesh). Following recent cuts in health budgets, the source of nurse recruits dramatically shifted from the industrialized countries to the developing countries in order to reduce the payroll and maintain staff numbers. The majority of nurses now recruited to the Middle East are from the Philippines, India, Sri Lanka, and sub-Saharan Africa, as well as Sudan, Egypt, Jordan, and Tunisia.

So great are changes in migration flows that a country like Ireland, traditionally known as a nurse exporting country, is now experiencing a critical shortage that it is trying to solve by importing nurses by the dozens from China, the Philippines, Jordan, Australia, South Africa, New Zealand, the United Kingdom, and even the United States.[8] The number of source countries generating nurses for export has greatly increased in the past two decades. At the same time, the past North–North movement is increasingly being replaced by nurses from the South going to the North.

Relatively large emigration flows creating severe gaps in services are not limited to developing countries. Over the years France, especially the border regions with Switzerland, has provided thousands of nurses to its neighbors. The city of Geneva recruits 300 nurses a year but the local nursing school produces only 50 new graduates annually. The remaining 250 come from elsewhere, usually its neighbor France. This has aroused some debate. The matter has gone all the way to the French National Assembly, where legislators recently denounced the "poaching" of nurses by Geneva as intolerable.[9] According to Urs Weyermann, secretary-general of the Swiss

Nurses Association, three thousand nurses graduate each year from the country's various nursing schools. The problem, he adds, is not educating nurses but maintaining them in active practice. This, Weyermann believes, is a major cause of the nursing shortage.[10] Although much of the media attention on the problem of nurse migration has pitted wealthy countries against poorer ones, it is interesting that the friction between these two industrialized countries generates much of the passion and many of the same issues voiced in discussions of the South–North "brain drain."

Anne Brissiaud, director of nursing in a French hospital near the Swiss border, explains that 120 of their 350 employed nurses leave yearly—half to work in Switzerland and the other half to retire or leave the profession.[11] Although Brissiaud acknowledges that the nurse shortage has always existed, she points out that it has greatly increased in recent years. In fact, the hospital was obliged to close a thirty-bed unit for lack of personnel. Having spent eleven thousand euros advertising all over France to recruit nurses, the hospital was frustrated when those that did come worked for only several months and then went to work in Switzerland for better pay. A new graduate is paid €1,400 in France while in Geneva the salary is more than twice as high (the equivalent of €3,600). In addition, working conditions are said to be better in Switzerland, allowing more time to develop interpersonal relations with patients. Thus the French border regions become a stepping-stone for nurses making their way to better pay and career opportunities in Switzerland.

To deal with the problem, government officials often advise their neighboring countries to exercise a self-restraint in their appetite for nurses that they would be unable to exercise at home. For example, the mayor of Gaillard, a border town in France, suggested that Geneva limit itself to a specified number of cross-border workers. Given the fact that the bilateral agreement creating complete freedom of movement between Switzerland and the European Union (including France) went into effect in June 2004, this solution hardly seems realistic. Moreover, the Geneva University Hospital has publicly stated that they will not jeopardize the quality of their services by limiting recruitment efforts to find essential staff. In an effort to recruit ethically, this hospital did voluntarily withdraw all vacancy ads from the local French papers. This, however, did not stop French nurses from responding to the recruitment ads that are routinely placed in the national professional journals (French and Swiss) or on the Internet.

In an attempt to compensate France for its reluctant contribution to the Swiss health care system, one of the Swiss nursing schools in the area proposed taking students from French secondary schools, thus participating in the cost of training future staff. Unwilling to spend the SF 24,000 in subsidies (per student for four years of education), Swiss politicians rejected this proposal. They preferred to maintain the status quo—recruiting more cheaply the already qualified nurses from abroad.

According to the newspaper *Le Temps,* there is one care provider for every six to eight patients in Switzerland, compared to one for eighty patients in the French communes neighboring Geneva.[12] While the numbers may not be quite as dramatic as the critical situations faced by many developing countries, it is amazing how the same concerns are voiced by industrialized and developing countries alike in this international war for skills. Similar arguments are made in each case, and parallels can be drawn between the various strategies recommended as well as the reasons given for their rejection.

International Migration of Professionals

Nurses have been clearly among the professionals most in demand during the years 1995–2005. Patricia Sto. Tomas, secretary of labor of the Philippines, refers to the exporting of nurses as the new growth area for overseas employment.[13] Whereas seamen and domestic workers used to dominate the Filipino migrant labor force, nurses are now a very profitable market niche and represent a principal wave of migrant workers.

For professional workers, the discrepancy between overseas wages and local salaries is usually greater than for unskilled workers. Professionals have a greater potential economic gain from migrating and are more interested in employment opportunities abroad. It is no wonder that they generally seek "to maximize return on their personal investment in education and training by moving in search of the highest paid and/or most rewarding employment."[14] They have many more options for overseas employment than a maid or unskilled laborer. Professionals are also more likely to be better informed of opportunities abroad and have greater access to financial resources needed to migrate.

Emigration is therefore selective. It focuses on "those who can afford it, whose skills are in demand abroad, and who stand to benefit most."[15] There is a widespread need for nursing skills, an industry eager to facilitate the movement of nurses to meet this demand worldwide, and professionals willing to consider employment opportunities abroad. All the factors are in place that encourage the mass migration of nurses around the world.

The most reliable global estimates on the international migration of professional workers are from the 1998 International Monetary Fund study. Since the data are from the 1980s, the findings reflect the pre-globalization era and are probably lower than the present-day figures. Nevertheless, among the 12.9 million documented skilled workers emigrating from developing countries, the rate was found to be highest among the very well educated (tertiary level), averaging about 30 percent from any single country.[16] According to Ajit Ghose, the average emigrant from developing countries had received twice as many years of education as the average inhabitant.[17] In other words, a minimum of one-third of the professionals educated in developing countries practice their skills elsewhere and may leave behind a vulnerable population with a threatened potential for economic growth. Thus we may have the problem of brain drain.

Brain Drain

Simply put, brain drain is a transfer of human capital from one country to another, much as traditional trade is a transfer of goods from one country to another.[18] Taking into consideration professionals' desire to maximize the investment in their education, brain drain has also been defined as "the emigration or flight of skilled human capital from one country to the other in search of better returns to one's knowledge, skills, qualifications and competencies."[19]

Neither of these definitions captures all the dimensions of the concept. For example, in situations where the source country has a surplus of skilled professionals, the term *brain drain* is rarely used. The fundamental essence of the term is associated with circumstances where professionals who are desperately needed in the source country decide to migrate. It suggests not just a limited migration but an outflow siphoning off a critical mass or significant number of professionals. This implies, of course, that source countries are deprived of a set of much-needed skills. But not just skills are lost. As mentioned, countries also lose on the investment of the funds they have spent on helping professionals develop these highly marketable skills through education and training. Fundamental to most debates on the brain drain, then, are the negative economic implications or the financial loss experienced by source countries, usually developing nations.

In addition to education and training expenses, we must also consider what are known as opportunity costs. What could have been achieved if these funds had been used differently?[20] What if wasted monies had been put to better use—for training someone who would have stayed in the source country and provided services, for example, or for improving the pay and working conditions of employed personnel, thus raising retention rates?

Finally, source countries lose the right to tax the higher incomes expected from graduates of tertiary education institutions. Since skilled workers earn three to ten times as much as unskilled workers, this significantly reduces government revenue that could eventually be reinvested in the sector for future generations of students.

The brain drain debates have spanned four decades. During this period their visibility has ebbed and flowed. In the 1960s and 1970s, the brain drain of skilled workers across the globe became a hot topic and then receded from public attention. With globalization, discussions of brain drain and the costs and benefits of migration resurfaced in the early 1990s and continue to this day. The highly emotional and derogatory tone of the term suggests acute sensitivities. When it comes to nurses, source countries and international observers sometimes resort to increasingly inflammatory rhetoric—using the words *poaching* and *looting* to describe their recruitment from developing countries by wealthier industrialized countries. Poor countries accuse richer ones of stealing their knowledge and skills in a kind of peculiar process of "reverse subsidy."[21] Some have gone as far as to invoke the history of Western colonial occupation, arguing that nurse migration is a new form of colonialism: with developing countries once again exploited.

What all this Sturm und Drang conceals is the fact that poorer countries are not entirely innocent victims of the voracity of their wealthier counterparts. Ironically, for example, inter-African migration may come very close to the volume of workers or asylum seekers knocking at the doors of industrialized countries.[22] Indeed, the reframing of the issue is fascinating. When African ministers talk about intraregional nurse migration, it is not usually referred to in terms of brain drain. Quite the opposite. African ministers talk of promoting intraregional exchanges of workers in the hope of encouraging economic growth for the whole region. Although flows between developing countries also deplete the source country's workforce, appeals to solidarity among equals play an important role in influencing the perception of migration. The destination country should not be relevant to the debate, and yet somehow it is. South-to-South migration may attract more attention in the coming years, however, as many fast-growing, newly industrialized countries in the South are expected to attract more migration than the industrialized countries.[23] Brain drain today continues to imply a migration flow from South to North, which tends to be the case for nursing where it is a source of greatest concern. Yet, we cannot ignore the fact that much of nurse migration takes place between highly developed countries, where nurses are supposed to have far greater opportunities.

There is no doubt that difficult working conditions, heavy workloads, and low ratios of qualified to assistant personnels only get worse when nurses emigrate—contributing to the push factors that characterize nurse

migration and ultimately affect the quality of care provided by the health facility and system as a whole. Cathy Andrews, a UK nurse now working in
Australia, provides a clear glimpse of these daily realities and describes the
frightening conditions that set the scene for overstretched health care providers. Andrews, an experienced nurse who had worked for many years in
the National Health Service, left the United Kingdom, she insists, most likely
forever. Her first and only stop so far has been Australia. Although she was
surprised by the fact that her salary was actually higher than she thought it
would be, her reason for leaving was less financial than professional. "I was
driven from the National Health Service because I could no longer cope with
the unrelenting grind," Andrews said regretfully. She continued,

> I could no longer cope with patient staffing levels of fifteen to one, with the
> nauseating, gut-wrenching, gnawing feeling that today was the day some-
> one might die because of me, because I had missed something. I could no
> longer cope with providing care as well as running the ward, sorting out sick-
> ness and absence, supervising junior staff and students, answering phones,
> dealing with relatives and being expected to provide displays, write infor-
> mation leaflets, study in my own time for no reward, and attend meetings
> where management neither understood nor cared about the opinions of their
> staff. I could no longer cope with not being able to spend time with grieving
> families and being told we were not to offer bereaved relatives cups of tea
> because of the cost. I could no longer cope with managers who threatened
> and bullied to appropriate funds that were set aside for patients and staff,
> many of which were charitable donations. I could not cope with 18-hour
> shifts because someone failed to turn up and managers expected staff to
> work late, then the night with no break. . . . I am tired of people speculating
> about why nurses leave, the reasons are plain.[24]

Andrews left an industrialized country and ended up in another affluent
nation. On the units she left behind, her disappearance would have been
sorely noted. The departure of nurses from active practice may have an even
more demoralizing and devastating effect in countries where hospitals and
health services are barely coping with the lack of personnel. Then the loss of
one or two staff with specialist skills may be more significant than the loss
of a greater number of unskilled workers. Martineau writes about the Centre for Spinal Injuries in Boxburg, South Africa. On the very same day in
2000, the center's two anesthetists were recruited to Canada. Unable to find
replacements, this referral center has been closed down ever since, affecting
the whole region.[25] The emigration of even a few professionals may mean
that patients are completely deprived of desperately needed services that
they will be unable to find elsewhere.

The excessive emigration of nurses affects the overall functioning of a health facility and leads to the depletion of a much-needed workforce. The number of patient deaths and of treatment or surgical complications increase. High turnover rates contribute to a substantial loss of institutional memory, which may result in a duplication of work and the wastage of resources. Inadequate supervision of assistant staff or new graduates deprives them of good role models and needed support, which, in turn, affects future generations of health care workers. The absence of sufficient nurse educators seriously threatens the quality of new nurse graduates, so the effects may be long term.[26] Beyond the hospitals or health centers, there may be gaps in the procurement of medicines or the management of epidemic threats to public health, for example SARS (severe acute respiratory syndrome). The brain drain affects all levels of the health system and is not limited to direct patient care.

Brian Chituwo, the health minister of Zambia, deplores the 50 percent nurse vacancy rate at the University Teaching Hospital, the country's largest health institution. The hospital requires a staff of fourteen hundred nurses, but only seven hundred are currently employed. Nurses are thus routinely asked to care for as many as forty patients instead of the recommended five. Chituwo told the press that about two thousand Zambian nurses are now in the United Kingdom, most of them working as maids. This, he said, is an incredible waste of urgently needed nursing skills. Zambia is now trying to address its brain drain. The government has raised nurses' salaries by close to 90 percent, has implemented rural hardship allowances, and has provided better housing for nurses. Dr. Chituwo is not, however, optimistic about the efficacy of these efforts. He understands that nurses have significant financial responsibilities—first of all, their obligations as salaried persons in the extended family, made even heavier these days by the increasing numbers of HIV/AIDS orphans. He worries that the remuneration offered in Zambia just cannot compete with salaries abroad.[27]

Janamitra Devan and Parth Tewari conclude that "the hard reality is that few emerging markets have any hope, in the foreseeable future, of creating the type and volume of economic opportunities needed to reverse or even substantially slow the brain drain."[28] While less than optimistic, this statement may be brutally helpful in generating a true overview of the situation and credible options to address the fundamental issues.

In discussions held at the World Health Assembly in May 2004, African ministers agreed that for the smallest countries in their region, with populations of less than one million, the loss of even one skilled health worker is significant. A health economist and an intensive care nurse trained in a small African country and then recruited to the United States represent an insignificant net gain of two health workers in this large human resources pool. On the other hand, the African country may have lost the last two key skilled staff in their respective areas, and they may be difficult to replace. The main thrust of a report submitted to the WHO executive board in May 2004 summarizes the challenges faced by many developing country health systems:

> Difficult working conditions, characterized by heavy workloads, lack of equipment, poor salaries and diminished opportunities for advancement, result in increased migration out of Africa, and, in countries, from the public to the private sector and from rural to urban areas. The net effect is to increase the workload of those who remain, especially in rural areas, where caring for disadvantaged people causes stress and demotivation, in turn encouraging even more professionals to migrate, and to decrease the quality of health care provided in institutions. The heavy workload on staff working in difficult conditions—in one country, the outpatient attendance-to-nurse ratio rose from 623 in 1995 to 963 in 2000 at district hospital level—results in long waiting times for patients. Furthermore, inequity in access to health care is increasing. Rural areas have always been disadvantaged, but, with loss of health workers, some health facilities no longer function or are run by unqualified staff.
>
> The quality of education has reportedly declined in nursing and midwifery schools owing to emigration of teaching staff, and the remaining trainers are unable to cope with the demand for the training and specialized programs of research needed in Africa. The quality of training and the capacity to provide evidence through research are thus compromised. Lack of supervision and mentoring is also a concern; senior, experienced staff are being lost through emigration.[29]

One nurse from Port Elizabeth wrote a letter to the editor of her professional journal in South Africa. Her description of nurses' anguish in dealing with extremely difficult daily situations dramatizes the message of the report.

> Many evenings we have a single nurse to care for a 45 bed ward and on many occasions the nurse is an Assistant Nurse. Bear in mind, this is a very busy referral hospital. One nurse may admit up to 10 patients per night. . . . At our hospital we often have three nurses to care for 90 patients! This is a medico-legal hazard on its own, but in extreme situations one registered nurse is allocated 145 patients per night! We have had many meetings with management, but to no avail. I think we're all on the verge of burn-out at our hospital. . . . We fetch treatments, commence intravenous antibiotics and attend to emergencies. The list is never ending. . . . They ask how you cope. I do not know. One thing I do know is that I cannot render effective patient care under these extreme conditions. I know transformation is in progress at our hospital, but every night is a risk while we are working like this.[30]

She signed the letter "Slavery," a clear indication of the moral burden and harsh working conditions nurses brave routinely.

The situation in the Caribbean is very similar. Although emigration data have not been systematically collected, what is available suggests that resignation from the public health system in order to follow job opportunities abroad has been the major contributor to the emerging nursing crisis.

The 2000 Trinidad and Tobago data reveal that "on average only every second nursing post is held by a professional nurse. The other half of the posts [are] either vacant or filled with retirees who came back to work on a part-time basis or with less qualified support staff. . . . Half to two thirds of all head nurses posts in the country were vacant."[31] One region of the country recorded particularly acute nursing shortages. The North Western Regional Health Authority in 2000 had on average two-thirds of all staff nursing posts vacant. The Caura Hospital was particularly hard hit. Although it remained open, only a quarter of all nursing posts were filled. At the community level, health services reported 30 percent shortage of nurses. These shortages severely limited the district health care facilities' ability to deliver needed services. In spite of the fact that no hard data prove the link between emigration and such drastic shortages, the Ministry of Health and its researchers firmly believe that emigration is the primary underlying reason. The implied link between shortages and emigration begs the question, If there was no emigration, would these rural health facilities be better staffed? Would more nurses be prepared to work there, or would they look for other options in an urban area or in the private sector?

The migration flows out of the Caribbean are not limited to nurses. They affect every level of the regional labor market. The fact remains that the region has lost more than five million people over the last fifty years. The trigger for the mass exodus of professionals is said to be the rising demand for highly qualified people in North America and the United Kingdom.

The Global Treasure Hunt

When describing the new nurse migration, researchers and other observers often invoke the image of a carousel or global treasure hunt to describe the migration flow from rural to urban centers, from poorer to wealthier urban neighborhoods, and then from poorer to wealthier countries.[32] The implication is that nurses will discover the treasure at the end of the hunt. That is not always the case. For many nurses, the search for a better life is not always successful. Nurses have migrated only to find that their quality of life, working conditions, and environment had not greatly improved. Janey Parris, formerly with the Commonwealth secretariat, confirms that "in due course the foreign nurses discover that while conditions of work are somewhat better than from where they have come, there are still numerous deficiencies with which they are unable to cope and before long they are gone."[33] As mentioned, because emigration is selective, appealing to the "migration prone," the global treasure hunt may go on indefinitely, with disappointed migrants moving again and again if they become disenchanted with their circumstances.[34]

Unhappy or disappointed migrant nurses may decide to close the circle and return home. Many, however, are conscious that the factors and circumstances that led them to migrate have not changed in their home countries. Equipped with more skills and knowledge—perhaps higher degrees—they may decide to try another foreign country where they will find better prospects for career satisfaction.

Again, none of these calculations are limited to nurses from developing countries. There has been extensive literature written on the brain drain from Canada to the United States. In a domino-like effect, professionals are then drawn from third countries—especially from developing countries—to Canada to make up the loss.[35] The OECD countries, as a group of industrialized and therefore wealthier nations, are considered true magnets for professional workers, including health professionals. The United States is repeatedly identified as the epicenter of international migration. Because it has the greatest ongoing need for skilled labor and the financial means to recruit widely, the United States exerts the strongest pull.

Global Productivity

The examples above emphasize the perspective of nation-states and individuals. Some economists look at international professional migration with a broader view. In the 1960s there was some consensus that "global welfare is raised by the rational choice of highly skilled emigrants to seek improved incomes abroad."[36] It seemed logical that if the number of persons with higher incomes increased, the general welfare of the world would also improve. The assumption was that the migrant Ghanaian nurse now working in England earns a higher salary. The world's revenue-generating potential has therefore been increased as a direct result of this nurse's increase in pay. The global gross domestic product, which includes the sum of all workers' earnings, will increase in an amount equivalent to the difference in wages between the past and present jobs.

When explored more closely, this seems to be an unrealistic conclusion.

Because it is so theoretical, it ignores many of the other factors that contribute to economic and social well-being. The local positive impact of an additional nurse in the destination country may not compensate for the potential negative impact in the source country of losing one of its health professionals.

On the other hand, productivity at the global level may increase as a result of international migration. An individual with potential but no resources will tend to be less productive than the same individual with the means to facilitate the delivery of products or services. Given the imperfect work environment in many developing countries, it is difficult for skilled professionals to work to their full potential. Qualified nurses capable of providing acute care services such as giving intravenous injections or taking electrocardiograms are severely limited if they are not provided with the necessary tools and materials. For example, the Community Working Group on Health in Zimbabwe reports that "rural clinics often lack electricity, food, bedclothes and even paper on which to record a patient's medical history."[37] Private clinics in the country tend to be better equipped but remain almost empty. Patients who cannot pay for the services are not allowed entry. The journalist Anne Wayne describes the scene. "Sick people huddle on the doorstep, as if hoping that the proximity to medicine will heal them. Inside, rows of empty beds are made up with fresh linen and nurses slump on stools, waiting in vain for a patient who can afford treatment. 'I feel so helpless,' said one nurse. 'You cannot treat people without tools and medicine.'"[38] This nurse's dilemma is all the more frustrating when the medicine is available but too expensive for patients. Even though their countries suffer from critical nurse shortages, nurses in these situations are underemployed.

Placing this nurse in an environment where there are sufficient resources, and where patients can access the materials, equipment, and care providers they need, will no doubt increase productivity at the individual as well as the global level. However, if maximum productivity depends on international migration, this increase brings little comfort to the patients that could benefit from nursing care in Zimbabwe.

It may also bring little consolation to some nurses whose skills are underutilized in the developed countries to which they have migrated. This deficient utilization of nurses' skills in industrialized countries, discussed in the previous chapters, creates the phenomenon known as "brain waste." "Highly qualified overseas-trained nurses arrive to find they are expected to carry out menial tasks. Some health professionals attempt to get registration in country, but end up as 'assistants' in their profession . . . working far below their potential."[39] One thirty-one-year-old Kenyan nurse now working in the United Kingdom expresses her grief and anguish: "Some of the skills I had—they're dead because I don't have a chance to use them."[40] It is a loss that the world cannot afford.

Underemployed or unemployed nurses in source countries may at times suffer from the same anguish, the same professional limitations, but for different reasons. There are cases of brain waste when nurses remain in their home country and fail to find employment. In countries like Tanzania, for example, there are no jobs for new graduates of nursing schools. Although Tanzania is suffering from a nursing shortage, even experienced nurses are unemployed. Because no budgeted or paid posts are available, these nurses volunteer to work for free in local hospitals. They do this because they fear losing their skills and the chance of getting future employment. Ironically, although half of all nursing positions in Kenya are unfilled, Volqvartz reports one third of all Kenyan nurses are unemployed. The modern paradox of shortage side by side with unemployment is difficult to grasp and often completely ignored by policy makers worldwide. Taking yet another example, Grenada's twenty-seven nurse graduates in 2004 found themselves unemployed after graduation. While the health system is barely coping with the strain of high vacancy rates, it cannot financially afford to absorb these willing nurses. In cases such as these, international migration may be a difficult but worthy option. Brain waste or de-skilling is a common threat to both destination and source countries—and an unacceptable reality in the light of the critical global shortages of nursing skills.

Beneficial Brain Drain

The neoclassical models of economic development and more recent economic theory (e.g., endogenous growth theory) tend to agree that high-skilled emigration reduces national economic growth rates. Research demonstrated that a one-year decrease in the average education of a nation's workforce decreases productivity levels by 5–15 percent.[41] The emigration of highly educated professionals will necessarily decrease the nation's average education levels. Taken in isolation, it is likely to have a negative impact on national productivity.

A certain amount of migration may, however, be beneficial and act as a stimulus to domestic education as well as business opportunities. Attractive career opportunities abroad tend to stimulate nationals to undertake further studies. Nurses admit that one of the profession's attractions is the knowledge that career opportunities await them abroad once they become qualified. The booming education sector in the Philippines is proof that training nursing professionals is a lucrative and growing business. This is also demonstrated by the various conversion courses and distance learning programs that the private sector in industrialized countries has generated to meet the demand for international nurse migrants. In many developing countries, up to 50 percent of the graduating class of nurses report their intention to work abroad. As mentioned earlier, there is ample evidence that the international recruitment of nurses is a growth industry in and of itself.

At a sufficiently high level of emigration, the proportion of skilled workers in a given country may increase. From their in-depth analysis of the data, B. Lindsay Lowell and Allan Findlay conclude that "the possibility of emigrating to higher wage countries may stimulate individuals to pursue higher education in anticipation of finding better-paid work abroad. . . . At a sufficiently high volume of skilled emigration, the share of skilled workers in the source country actually grows."[42] The promising career opportunities abroad act as a marketing or promotion message for young and mature adults to enter a given profession. The case of lawyers and physicians becoming nurses demonstrates this trend. Striking the correct balance between new graduates and the rate of emigration will support the maintenance or expansion of an active workforce. Beyond this optimal rate, however, the depletion of the skilled workforce occurs too quickly for the critical mass of national professionals to be maintained.[43] These societal responses imply that some migration is necessary or beneficial for development. The critical factor in determining the net result and impact of brain drain is therefore a matter of degree. When is enough, enough? When do the disadvantages outweigh the benefits? Is it possible for brain drain to be transformed into brain gain in both source and destination countries? Are there opportunities for mutual benefit?

Brain Gain

There is no doubt that destination countries benefit from the international migration of nurses. These skilled professionals fill critical gaps in services. They often accept positions that local nurses refuse—posts in rural, isolated communities; shifts that are less popular; service areas that are sometimes considered less attractive or inappropriately stigmatized—for example, care of the elderly. Studies show that recruited personnel tend to settle in more rural, underserved, high need, and deprived areas. Hawthorne's data from Australia showed the disproportionate concentration of foreign nurses with non-English-speaking backgrounds in the "least prestigious nursing home sector—a sector in the process of redefinition as for 'foreign labor.'"[44] The reality of such high proportions of migrant professionals in this sector has dramatically modified its image. People quickly assume that foreign personnel will agree to staff these workplaces. Do we run the risk of having these jobs doubly stigmatized—first because they are too difficult, too remote, or too low tech, and then again because it is work only foreigners will do?

The implementation of an immigration policy requiring foreign professionals to work in predetermined areas is now being investigated in at least one country as a violation of human rights. This may not be relevant for nursing. In general, recruits are directed toward vacant posts and a significant percentage of them tend to be in areas rejected by local employees.

The facilitated or fast-track visa processes that some industrialized countries have introduced may, however, favor a more forcefully directed migration channel. In the United States, for example, the H-1C visa, created by the Nursing Relief for Disadvantaged Areas Act of 1999, specified federally designated health professional shortage areas where hospitals were eligible to apply for the H-1C visa. By March 2002, only fourteen hospitals nationwide had met the Department of Labor's requirements for these visas.[45] While the numbers were small (a maximum of five hundred such visas were allowed per year), and the offer time limited (the act expired in August 2004), similar initiatives are being developed by other industrialized countries desperate to supplement the local labor market with foreign nurses.

Migrant nurses have tended to be categorized as less assertive, more flexible, less demanding, and often more respectful of authority, especially those coming from Asia. Partly, this is attributed to their more vulnerable employment situation as foreigners; partly, to their culture and education. According to the American Nurses Association, "many employers know that foreign-educated nurses will not speak up about poor working conditions or unfair treatment."[46] In 2003, for example, the *New York Times* did a long article on the virtues of Filipino nurses. In it, Diane Aroh, the chief nurse executive of Montefiore hospital, said she valued her Filipino nurses not only because they are very compassionate but also because "they're very flexible, willing to take new assignments on the spur of the moment, willing to work extra-long hours."[47]

After undertaking a decades-long study on nurses in the Philippines, Irma Bustamante said she found that altruism is part of their nature. They have been socialized to render service without expecting anything in return. This, she believes, is one of the reasons why nurses do not assertively fight for their rights.[48] All of this, of course, can bring short-term advantages for employers who may appreciate having a flexible, compliant, less unionized, and more loyal or dependent workforce. In situations of labor conflict, newly recruited migrant nurses tend to be less involved in industrial actions such as strikes. Employers in nonunionized facilities, especially in private-sector environments, often push wages down, as they did in the Texas, California, and UK cases presented in chapter 3.

Yet, there is no denying the valuable and needed contributions made by nurses from abroad. One English nurse acknowledges the positive experience of working with migrant nurses: "I feel very privileged to work with such compassionate and knowledgeable people, and to be given the chance to learn about life and attitudes in different parts of the world. Without foreign nurses, some of our hospitals would not be able to cope with the demands made on them, and people would not receive the care they need. The burden on existing nurses such as myself would be intolerable, and any joy or satisfaction from nursing would disappear under an increasing mountain of work."[49]

Other nurses in host countries recognize that migrant nurses help them deal with an increasingly multicultural patient population. The advantages of having a transcultural nursing team and care approach are self-evident. Nurses from other cultures may demonstrate a greater respect of patients' cultural backgrounds. They may have greater knowledge of their health expectations and an understanding of their health beliefs—all fundamental building blocks of a credible nursing/patient care plan. Plus, they may share with patients a common language, which is, of course, an essential prerequisite to communication. What is so ironic about this benefit of nursing migration is the fact that so few industrialized societies make use of the skills of previous generations of migrants in their standard domestic recruiting. The nursing workforce in many industrialized countries tends to be monocultural, with ethnic minorities essentially ignored as a potential pool of new recruits. So, for example, the US health care system has spent little time recruiting from the Jamaican-American community but eagerly recruits in Jamaica. Similarly, there are growing Chinese migrant populations in many of the industrialized countries, including the United States and the United Kingdom. They have been generally ignored as a potential pool of students who could become locally trained nurses. And yet China is now considered a new source country for already qualified nurses.

According to the 2000 Census Bureau figures, 12.1 percent of the resident population of the United States were black (non-Hispanic) and another 12.5 percent were Hispanic.[50] The differences are striking when considering the registered nurse population of the United States. In March 2000 only 5.1 percent of the registered nurses were black (non-Hispanic) and 2.2 percent Hispanic.[51] The race/ethnic group that compared favorably was the Asian population—0.7 percent and 3.8 percent respectively. Given that the largest group of imported nurses is from the Philippines, this suggests that in fact the majority of these nurses are foreign educated and not "homegrown." In contrast, white non-Hispanics represent 86 percent of the nurse population and only 70 percent of the resident population.

Because of the new nursing shortage the mind-set is slowly changing. In industrialized nations, there is now greater effort to attract ethnic minorities and men to join the ranks of nursing. While this is not directly related to international migration, it does indicate that health systems are more open to accepting staff from a multitude of backgrounds and are actively promoting diversity among health professionals. For example, Tenet Healthcare Corporation operates thirty hospitals in southern California, where more than 40 percent of its patients but only 4 percent of the health care professionals are of Latino descent. The Tenet Healthcare Foundation's grant of $1 million to provide financial support to Latino nursing students is one attempt to adjust the ethnic balance of the workforce to more closely parallel the population as a whole.

Caution is needed when considering ethnic balance. Data just released from the Center for Health Workforce Studies demonstrate that while foreign-born nurses dramatically increase the diversity of the US nurse workforce, they do not necessarily serve the same cultures from which they come. If most Asian nurses in a community are Filipino, for example, while most of the residents are Chinese, cultural competence is far from guaranteed. Jean Moore and colleagues argue that regional as opposed to cultural representation is misleading and may weaken equal-opportunity recruitment campaigns targeting ethnic groups within the local population.[52]

The Pan-American Health Organization estimates the total loss of government investments to educate nurses to the basic level, and then have them emigrate, to be about $16.7 million per year for the Caribbean.[53] The expense of educating health professionals is significant. Tremendous savings result for the destination country (taken as a whole) when public monies from other countries cover these education costs. According to the Healthcare Association of New York State, it costs only $10,000 to $12,000 to hire a foreign nurse and bring her to the United States for active employment in nursing.[54] As mentioned earlier, savings reach into the billions. Which is why so many developing countries demand that industrialized countries compensate them for their loss of skilled professionals and the money invested in educating them.

Given the multiple routes to nursing education, the many ways this education is financed, and the complex career paths taken by nurses, it will be very difficult to create any credible or equitable compensation system as part of a bilateral or multilateral governmental agreement. Three main factors are at the hub of the debate: the duration of the migration, the portion of the education costs that are to be compensated, and the public or private nature of the destination country employment.

Imagine, for example, Nurse Clarke[†] from Ghana. Public finances allocated to the Ministry of Education paid for her primary and secondary schooling. The Ministry of Health financed her three-year tertiary nursing education program. As a student, she provided nursing services in hospital and community facilities operated by the Ministry of Health. After graduation, she accepted a job in the United Kingdom to work in a privately owned nursing home. To qualify for employment, she had to go through a three-month adaptation or supervised practice program. It took her one year to be officially registered as a professional nurse. Without her official registration, she could only find work as a nursing assistant at a considerably lower salary. At the beginning of her second year in the United Kingdom, she decided to transfer to the public health service and worked in the cardiology unit of an acute care hospital. Clarke was not happy with the work environment. So she got back on the carousel and decided to migrate to a developing country, South Africa, to be closer to her family and traditions. After several years there, she decided it was time to return home.

This example illustrates the complex path taken by many migrant nurses. With all these variables and more, any compensation system would be a labyrinth of rules, regulations, and exceptions. Very sophisticated national and international registries and databases would need to be established. It is an understatement to say that they do not yet exist, and perhaps a fantasy to believe they could. Emigration and immigration records would have to be updated daily, requiring human and financial resources not easily available. Invoicing and banking systems permitting the transfer of funds in a timely and reliable manner would also be needed. The cost of operating such a system would probably be so prohibitive as to be counterproductive.

Nevertheless, there continues to be a call for such a reparation system from the developing countries faced with the continual loss of public funds and local investment potential. In 2004 some African ministers of health once again raised the matter at the World Health Assembly (WHA), the supreme decision-making body of the World Health Organization. Their wish was to develop ways to compensate for the loss of skilled health professionals from developing countries and the investment made in their training. The discussion between developed and industrialized countries was tense, which is understandable considering the sums of money implicated. Several open consultations were held and a small drafting committee was established to revise the WHA resolution enabling the organization and its members to address the issues in a coherent manner.

The minister of health of South Africa categorized the international migration of health personnel as "an international emergency" that needed to be addressed globally. The minister of health of Ghana added that the current migration was of epidemic proportions and that as a result the "human capacity for meeting the Millennium Development Goals was not there." The perspectives of the industrialized world were expressed by representatives from the European Union, the United States, Canada, and Australia, who emphasized the benefits of migration for both developed and developing countries.

Many of the participants from the developing countries agreed with the Barbados representative who spoke of seamless or free-flowing migration being the natural result of globalization and acknowledged that remittances from emigrants were a major financial asset. The African representatives argued that migration has some positive effects but that there is an urgent need to mitigate its negative impact. The impracticalities of a financial compensation system were, however, highlighted. The representative from Kenya acknowledged that his country was losing thirty experienced nurses every month. Unexpectedly, he added, "We're not asking you to send them back, only help us train more." (But will they be trained only to leave as soon as they graduate? That issue was studiously ignored.)

The language of the WHA resolution was in fact changed to reflect this dialogue, and emphasis was given to staff-retention measures and strengthening health systems rather than developing a financial compensation system. The resolution, accepted by consensus, sets out ambitious tasks for the coming years. For example, member states are urged to "establish mechanisms to mitigate the adverse impact on developing countries of the loss of health personnel through migration, including means for the receiving countries to support the strengthening of health systems, in particular human resources development, in the countries of origin."[55] The WHO director-general is assigned eleven major tasks to support the member states in managing migration, including reporting back at the 2005 and 2006 World Health Assembly.

The Commonwealth Code of Practice for the International Recruitment of Health Workers takes a similar track and bypasses any mention of a direct payment system. The code's Companion Document further clarifies the concept of compensation:

> Many developing Commonwealth countries have expressed the view that recruiting developed countries should in some way compensate source countries for the loss of personnel they have trained at great expense. Compensation may be in a variety of ways, such as building capacity in training institutions and reinsertion training. Compensation could also take the form

of arrangements which would include the provision of training programs. Such training should be relevant to the context of the source country so that the difficulties and frustration experienced by returning recruits are minimised. There could be more general programs to reciprocate for the recruitment of a country's health workers through the transfer of technology, skills and financial assistance to the country concerned.[56]

The Southern African Development Community in its 2001 statement also avoids any mention of direct financial compensation. While labeling the recruitment of their nurses by developed countries as "looting," they urge the application of the Commonwealth Code, capacity building assistance, the formalization of international recruitment through bilateral agreements, and the use of development funding to improve the conditions of service of their health workers.[57] Innovative methods of reparation are being sought, and the discussion may turn out to be more constructive and practical.

Under the current system, destination countries like the United Kingdom, the United States, and Canada, among others, are clearly saving money recruiting health professionals abroad. In the United Kingdom, "although the cost of hiring nurses from overseas is typically £2,000–£4,000, this is generally less than the costs of advertising, temporary replacements and appointment costs for experienced home-grown nurses, which the United Kingdom Department of Health has estimated at about £40,000."[58]

In countries where nurse education is primarily private, these considerations may not be as relevant. Governments have, however, addressed the challenge of nursing and financial shortages by introducing major increases in scholarships and student loans to support the expansion of the current pool of student nurses. Even when the private education sector is largely responsible for nursing education, public monies are used to subsidize institutions and support students.

From the source countries' perspective, there are also some advantages to the migration of nurses to wealthier countries. Brain drain may morph into brain gain under certain conditions.

Brain Drain to Brain Gain

If they maintain ties with their homelands, migrant nurses can offset the negative consequences of brain drain. One important contribution, already discussed, is the transfer of savings earned in the destination country. The International Organization for Migration reports that globally, these remittances represent a major source of hard currency (especially for the least developed countries) and make often substantial contributions to gross domestic product (GDP). In 2000, remittances sent by the diaspora to El Salvador, Eritrea, Jamaica, Jordan, Nicaragua and Yemen enabled these countries to augment their respective GDP by more than 10%. These resources allow foreign goods to be imported and national production to be strengthened. At the micro-economic level, remittances reinforce household revenues and are frequently used to purchase consumer goods or services. . . . [At the macro-economic level] they increase the total purchasing power of a given economy.[59]

In some countries, like Tonga, remittances account for as much as 39 percent of their GDP. According to a recent ILO study in Senegal, remittances constitute the principal source of household income—almost 90 percent—for those households that receive them.[60] This highlights the substantive dependence on remittances for family survival and security, not to mention the education of future generations.

Assuming that the migrant nurse will send money home, some families willingly and actively participate in covering the expenses of the initial migration because they know that their investment will be recovered and additional funds sent home will meet daily living expenses or education costs of relatives. Tim Martineau and his colleagues describe a Ghanaian father who took a sackful of money down to the Ministry of Health to pay off his daughter's bond. This liberated her from enforced government service and allowed her to find better-paid employment abroad as a nurse. The father was clearly confident that the family would be quickly reimbursed from her savings.[61] The available data documenting remittance flows (especially using informal channels of transfer), their impact, or the remittance behavior of various groups of migrant workers are either patchy or nonexistent. What we do know suggests that the transfer of savings from abroad is a tremendous support for many households and a valid stimulus for economic development of the source country.

Most developing countries need help from family members who work abroad. This need may be so dire that it conflicts with a country's need to retain skilled professionals at home. In the case of nurses, these conflicting priorities may be exacerbated by the fact that diverse government ministries may be directly involved and competing for the benefits produced. For example, a ministry of finance or foreign affairs may see the advantage of an incoming financial flow and closer links with other countries as the primary goal. On the other side of the street, the ministry of health may focus on the workforce shortages and gap in services that will result from the emigration of health professionals.

The total sum of remittances varies between data sources. According to the United Nations Conference on Trade and Development, the officially recorded global remittances weighed in at $117 billion in 2001 and are expected to increase yearly.[62] Incorporating remittances sent by unofficial channels, this figure can be doubled or tripled. In chapter 3 we saw how businesses benefit from the large sums of money migrant nurses send home. In African countries, with the exception of Nigeria and Cameroon, remittances far surpass foreign direct investment. The International Organization for Migration predicts that remittances will soon be twice as large as foreign aid and may be at least as effective in targeting the poor in both conflict-ridden and stable developing countries.[63] In the light of this financial dependence on the diaspora, any attempt to reduce international migration may have serious negative impact not only on families but also on the economic growth of developing countries.

While highly skilled migrants usually send a smaller share of their income, the likelihood that money will be sent home, and the absolute amount sent, increases with the emigrant's earnings.[64] This implies that professionals will send significant amounts of money back to their families, thus increasing the purchasing power not only of relatives but also of the nation.

The impact of all of this cash will depend on how the funds are used. In most cases, the families receiving help from abroad use the money for direct and immediate consumption purposes: food, housing, clothing, and education. This improves the health of the recipient families and, indirectly, their potential contribution to the national economy. If people are healthier, they can work more productively and earn more. When the money they earn and the remittances they receive are spent on local products and services, this will stimulate productivity, encourage job creation, and possibly increase local wages.

On the other hand, reliance on money from abroad can lead to growing dependence on foreign sources of income that may suddenly disappear if foreign economies no longer need as many migrant laborers. Remittance flows are necessarily affected by the economic cycles of destination countries, increasing when times are good, decreasing when poor. Even with cyclical swings, the amount of remittances is remarkably stable and, in fact, more reliable than private capital (business investment) flows.[65] Because remittances depend as much on the altruism of the workers who generate them as on the economies in which they work, when families are faced with particularly severe hardships in the source countries the flow of money transferred may actually increase.

Among economists who debate the issue there is no consensus on whether remittances, by themselves, cover or exceed the losses incurred by the source country when its professionals emigrate. One empirical analysis of remittances to Eastern Europe concluded that they do not offset the reduction in economic growth due to the loss of human capital.[66] Dilip Ratha, on the other hand, states that remittances more than offset the loss of tax revenue in most developing countries. Furthermore, when compared to domestic remittances (urban workers sending savings to relatives living in rural areas), international remittances have a more positive impact on savings and investment. The propensity to save is higher, and these funds are more often used as insurance policies associated with new production or entrepreneurial activities.[67]

Where countries are faced with the unemployment or underemployment of nurses, emigration represents a clear net gain for the source country. If there is a surplus of nurses—as is the case in Colombia, where 38 percent of nurses are unemployed—it is obviously cheaper to encourage them to work abroad than to provide them with unemployment or other social security benefits. This would also apply in industrialized countries with a surplus of nurses, whether long-term or of a temporary nature (as in Spain and Finland).

One study focusing on Filipino physicians practicing overseas concluded that the money they sent home more than compensated for the economic losses associated with their departure.[68] Similarly, John Connell and Richard Brown found that the remittances of migrant Tongan and Samoan nurses substantially exceeded the cost of their training and have contributed to raising standards in those countries.[69] This study, which specifically focused on nurses, found that as an occupational group they are more likely to send money home—and to send larger amounts—than other migrants. Why? For the usual reasons: Nurses tend to be more altruistic, and because they are predominantly female, they tend to be more reliably concerned about the family they have left behind. Recent research on Caribbean nurses found that 83 percent of the respondents sent remittances home to their families, and 26 percent were able to transfer more than half of their earnings.[70]

Once family survival is assured, remittances are often used for material benefits and local investments that stimulate economic growth. Migrant professionals are more likely to invest in their home countries. They invest in their uncle's small business, buy a second home, send a cousin to school.[71] Though they may live thousands of miles away, migrant nurses tend to maintain close ties with their family. Some make frequent visits to their homelands or prepare to return there sooner or later.

In Dennis Brown's study of migrant and nonmigrant Caribbean nurses, 40 percent of the migrants were homeowners before migrating; the figure rose to 70 percent after their emigration and return. Business owners moved from 5 percent to 14 percent, and car owners went from 37 percent to 63 percent. Among the nurse respondents who had never emigrated, only 32 percent owned a car, 24 percent owned a home and none owned a business.[72] The significant advantage of working abroad is clear for many nurses and their families. In terms of real estate, construction jobs, and material purchases, they contribute to the local economy. Indeed, their relative financial success may set local expectations of nurses and promote future emigration.

Nicholas Stern of the World Bank recently commented, "Nine-tenths of investment in developing countries comes from domestic sources."[73] A significant percentage of these domestic funds may be from remittances. For example, studies estimate that one-fifth of the capital invested in microenterprises in urban Mexico come from the remittances sent from the United States.[74]

Some doubt has been expressed as to the actual impact of remittances on the health sector. While there are indirect effects (improved standard of living for the receiving relatives), the funds may not often find their way back into education or health services. There are many reports that remittances have been used to build schools and clinics, but the numbers may not be high enough to make a significant impact on the sectors as a whole. Governments are increasingly creating investment possibilities specifically designed to channel remittances to priority public projects. Links with the diaspora are essential for such initiatives to be successful, and these are being nurtured through direct communication network structures, for example, the Internet. At least forty-one new e-based expatriate networks were established during the 1990s.[75] These are potentially very useful mechanisms to maintain links, channel information, stimulate research or entrepreneurial projects, and nurture partnerships.

In developing countries, workers' remittances have become such an important source of economic security and stability that they are part of a remarkable new economic development. Underscoring their value and reliability, in some countries economic remittances are now being offered as collateral for the creation and launch of bonds on the global investment market. Using the promise of future benefits (or future-flow receivables) as collateral has traditionally been the practice for oil exports or future generations of cattle. Some countries are now focusing on the use of remittances as an absolute value and reliable collateral—essentially taking out a loan with the promise to pay back with money collected from their migrant workers in the future. For example, "in August 2001 Banco do Brasil issued $300 million worth of bonds (with five-year maturity) using as collateral future yen remittances from Brazilian workers in Japan. . . . Developing country issuers could potentially raise about $7 billion a year using future remittance-backed securitization."[76] Mexico has the distinction of being the first country in the world to introduce future flows securitization—the creation of securities (stock-traded instruments) using future specific financial assets, including remittances, from abroad as collateral. The US$ Clearing Master Trust (Banorte) and US$ Diversified Payment Rights Master Trust (Banamex) are rated AA and AAA (i.e., highly reliable) investments.[77] In addition to Brazil and Mexico, El Salvador, Panama, and Turkey have used future workers' remittance-backed securities to increase external financing.

The realization that many migrant workers are putting their hard-earned money in bank accounts and using banking services for a charged fee has raised the interest of bankers all over the world. Attempts to attract more savings and generate more income-generating services are receiving greater attention. Foreign currency accounts are being encouraged to promote flows of external finances and remittances, offering prime rates of exchange and assured interest rates.

Imagine Nurse Ridder[+] from Curacao now working in the Netherlands. She receives her weekly salary in cash. After paying her bills and setting aside an amount for her incidental expenses, some money remains. Ridder needs to keep some cash for local emergencies and the rest she wants to send home. Her next visit to the family, however, will be in one year, and the relatives need the cash now. It is logical for Ridder to explore the options offered by the local banks and select the best deal. This may include a savings account with good interest rates or a bank transfer service charging an exceptionally low fee or a package deal between the Netherlands bank and a bank in Curacao that allows the transferred money to remain in euros, thus protecting her from the high inflation rate that exists in her home country.

Banking systems are paying more attention to this growth area and targeting new services to meet the needs of migrant workers. The PNB Trust Banking Group, based in the Philippines, for example, offers its Dollar Punla Fund, which it claims is a US dollar–denominated common trust fund geared for the overseas Filipino workers, where their small savings are pooled together and invested in high-grade US dollar–denominated financial instruments available locally and in other foreign financial markets.[78]

As mentioned, promoting the formal transfer of remittances provides a direct benefit to the banks. This is a high-margin business estimated to generate $12 billion in fees annually.[79] Governments, however, also benefit: they collect tax revenues from these services. Attempts to have a marketing edge in this growing transfer business has led to online services and remittances sent with personal messages for the recipient. Remit2India.com claims to be "the only door-to-door service available for remitting money to India. You can log in from the comfort of your office or home, and complete the transaction. The money is delivered directly to the door of your beneficiary via a locally payable Demand Draft or it is directly credited into the account in India. . . . You can follow the status of your remittance online on your 'Online Tracker' or just check your mailbox for e-mails from us updating you on every step of your transactions. . . . You can include a special personalized message to your beneficiary with every remittance, free of cost!"[80] Improving the formal remittance channels will tempt consumers to contract their services and generate income for a multitude of commercial enterprises along the way.

The diaspora not only stimulates innovations in services but also generates trade in goods from their source countries to the places they have chosen to relocate. To some extent, migrants tend to reproduce their home environment in their destination countries. Familiar foods, certain styles of clothing, reading materials in the native language—they all represent a market for import and export. To witness the value and dynamism of this kind of international exchange, one has only to walk down the streets of Queens or Notting Hill, where block after block of Korean or Indian groceries, video outlets, bookstores, and clothing shops alternate with a seemingly endless supply of exotic restaurants. One Canadian study concluded that a 10 percent increase in the number of immigrants from a given country was associated with a 1 percent increase in exports to that country and a 3 percent increase in imports.[81]

Remittances—cash, goods, and investments—are not the only transfers made by the diaspora to their source countries. There is also the vital transfer of ideas, information, and technology, as well as encouragement to take up collaborative projects. Hong Li, assistant professor of nursing at the University of Rochester, is part of a Chinese-American team of researchers on a nursing project unprecedented in China. After working seven years as a staff nurse at a Beijing Hospital, Li visited the Oregon Health Science University. What was to be a one-year visit was extended to pursue educational and research opportunities unavailable in China. Armed with a bachelor's, master's, and doctoral degree, she has become an expert in the care of the elderly. With another associate professor, Li has launched a comparative study investigating issues surrounding care for the elderly in US hospitals and comparing these results to hospitals in China.[82] Since there are more than 130 million people over the age of sixty in China, Li's contribution to the knowledge pool of her home country is guaranteed.

Brain Circulation

Due to major gaps and weaknesses in the available data, it is very difficult to quantify brain drain, globally or for specific countries. In fact, some experts are even questioning if it exists. Brain drain, which implies a loss to the source country of vital skills, professional knowledge, and management capacity, is relevant as a concept only if it is linked with permanent migration. If migrants return to their home country (or the country that has invested in their education), they will once again be a national resource, perhaps an enriched resource if acquired skills and knowledge are put to good use. Conclusive data are lacking. Many observers, however, believe that the return rate is quite high—at least 50 percent of skilled emigrants return from most stints (average 5 years) abroad.[83] So perhaps we should dispense with the term *brain drain* altogether and introduce a new concept, *brain circulation*. When considering health professionals, several researchers have documented that the rate of return for nurses is higher than for physicians.[84] The concept of brain circulation is therefore particularly relevant for nurses.

How does brain circulation work? As studies from the Caribbean demonstrate, migration is an integral part of the region's development process. One of its characteristics is circular flow. For example, Dennis Brown interviewed eighty Jamaican nurses, who had immigrated to the United States to work and had returned to their home country. Among these nurses, 24 percent had traveled abroad to work at least five times. Another 20 percent had gone abroad to work on at least six occasions. Eighty-eight per cent of these nurses now working in Jamaica intend to travel abroad again. Other stories and reports have documented that many Jamaican nurses seem almost to commute between Jamaica and the United States, where they work for very short periods or take on consecutive short-term assignments.[85] Of course, this kind of commuting between the Caribbean and the United States is far easier than that between the Philippines and London. But as international travel gets faster and easier, it may facilitate such work patterns for certain geographically close countries.

Responding to nurses' oft-repeated wish to have personal and professional experiences abroad, some entrepreneurial initiatives have offered employment that includes short periods of work abroad. The example of Netcare has already been given—complete teams of health care professionals from South Africa working for short periods of time to provide a specific service, cataract surgery, in the United Kingdom for the National Health Service. While the contracts with the foreign private health care provider, in this case Netcare, are long-term ones, the actual personnel spend only short periods abroad and are contractually obligated to return to the source country. Firms in Germany have also accepted UK contracts to provide periodic but short-term services in treatment centers newly established by the NHS.

One Swedish company has been providing teams of traveling health professionals supplying highly sophisticated renal dialysis care in the South Pacific islands. Faced with the difficulty of retaining specialists on the island, Samoa finds it more cost-effective to hire foreign teams that deliver a complete service (including maintenance of the equipment) and leave once it is provided. These generally for-profit initiatives are adaptations of past altruistic efforts of health professional teams traveling by boat to provide services to remote islands or coastal communities in developing countries.

The desire to work in a foreign country is not limited to qualified nurses but also includes nursing students. An increasing number of education programs incorporate periods of study abroad as a marketing attraction for potential students, highlighting the promising learning advantages. For example, in order to offer interesting internships for nursing students Monash University, Australia has established links with several UK hospitals.[86] In 2002 eighty students applied for six to eight clinical practice placements.

These experiences abroad are not limited to partnerships between universities based in industrialized countries. Students at Penn Nursing, a school at the University of Pennsylvania, are urged to explore a full range of options for study abroad. The Hebrew University of Jerusalem offers a program for third-year students that includes a clinical component in nursing care of childbearing families and nursing of children. Fieldwork based at Mahidol University School of Nursing in Thailand provides an intensive historical, sociopolitical, and cultural perspective on health and health care delivery, while the University of Hong Kong offers a comparative view of aging, public health, and allopathic, traditional, and complementary treatments.[87]

Clearly, nursing students, whether from developing or industrialized countries, are interested in exploring different health and sociopolitical realities. Greater understanding of other societies can only support advances in providing services to an increasingly multicultural patient population.

Migration flows and the potential for return migration depend on various factors. Many migrants wish to return but are met with bureaucratic obstacles and, at times, the absence of interesting job opportunities. In some developing countries experience abroad is accepted as part of the normal career path; it becomes a matter of prestige and may be considered a necessity for promotion (especially in academic circles). Some returning nurses, however, may discover that their coworkers are jealous because they have not had the same sorts of opportunities. Bimal Ghosh finds that many migrant returnees "are discouraged by the absence of a congenial environment to use their skills and resources and are disillusioned because of the lack of support from local and national authorities or by the negative attitude of the local community, including, not infrequently, its leaders."[88] Surprisingly, going home may add a financial burden for the returnees, since communities and family members expect them to display their "success" by making generous donations to community projects, throwing lavish banquets, and financing local fiestas.[89]

Migrant nurses who left the public service and were refused a leave without pay may face serious problems when they return home. Coming back with newly acquired skills, returning nurses expect to apply them in their new work environment and have these credentials recognized and justly rewarded. Rather than being greeted with open arms and put to work in areas that best utilize their new skills, many find that they are demoted. They receive lower salaries, lose any accrued benefits, and are denied prestige and professional recognition. Some find it impossible to secure a job at an appropriate level within the health system. Certain employers, particularly the more rigid public-sector services, make it difficult for former employees to rejoin the workforce.[90] The return migrant's only reward may be a different form of the frustration and dissatisfaction that led them to leave in the first place.

While the transfer of acquired skills is one of the potential benefits of return migration, there is no evidence that this actually occurs. It is unlikely that "a Zambian nurse working in an intensive care unit in the US will be able to transfer useful skills if she returns to a district hospital in her country."[91] It is not necessarily that her skills are not wanted or needed; it may be that the technology and other resources they require are simply not available. Depending on the rigidity of the workforce structures, returning nurses will either find employment that uses newly acquired skills, accept employment that ignores these skills, create a job within the structure, or branch out as an entrepreneur that puts these skills to advantage. There are also other options—leaving the health service or going abroad once again.

Many problems complicate the migrant's return. It is not easy to find employment opportunities at home when you are thousands of miles away. Information about job vacancies is hard to come by. The nurse who was disaffected enough to migrate will not want to return to just any job and will have to spend a lot of time finding what she considers to be just the right job. Florence Stephens is a good example of this complex process of reentry. A fifty-five-year-old UK-registered nurse and midwife, she reports being in excellent health after working in Saudi Arabia and the United Arab Emirates for twenty years and has stellar references. She returned to Wales, her native country, and then moved to London to find employment. Although the National Health Service is ostensibly crying out for highly qualified, experienced nurses, Stephens is not working in any of the hundreds of London hospitals. Instead, she is presently working for an agency, accepting temporary work until she finds permanent employment. After being refused two jobs in the National Health Service, the bureaucratic process has her baffled. "Prospective employers will not accept references from agencies. I have satisfactory references from my previous employment," says Stephens, "but in order to get a permanent job now, I need a reference from a present employer—but not an agency."[92] Stephens is so frustrated that she is even thinking of embarking on a new career, one that has nothing to do with nursing.

It does not seem possible that in a time of critical nursing shortages, such examples can coexist with massive international recruitment. Or that a foreign nurse can find the health care system in their new home helpful, while a native-born nurse is so frequently rebuffed. But this is one of the paradoxes of nurse migration—offering benefits to one nurse while seeming to withdraw them from another. All of this makes migration an enormous gamble.

Clearly, many of those who return do so after having significantly improved their financial status. While away, they may have used their savings to buy homes and establish businesses, either for themselves or for family members. As a result, their future is likely to be more secure. Others learn that economic development in their home countries now offers better opportunities than those that were available when they decided to go abroad. Young professionals are returning to the Caribbean from the United States since the modest economic recovery in the islands. Because of the economic recession in the United States, there is now less of a gap between the two economies.[93] Economic and political stability is important not only for encouraging foreign investment. It is also critical for bringing migrant workers back home.

The sense of change, particularly change for the better, is critical if return migration is to occur. Fatima Ansari organized a holiday visit back to the Middle East and was willing to consider a permanent return to her native country. When she found that nothing had changed, that all the reasons for her initial migration were still there, she went back to Sweden, her adopted home. "I was so looking forward to my first vacation back home," says Ansari. "I was even considering the possibility of returning permanently. My friends there told me I was crazy. I will never go back," she concludes.

Migration may follow distinct patterns depending on the source and destination country. When the cultures of both are very different, there is a tendency for migrant workers to take temporary employment and return to their native countries. Differences in family and social structure also play a fascinating role in the migration patterns of female nurses. For example, South African nurses tend to leave their children with the extended family when they work abroad and return once they have earned enough to meet their financial needs. They do so because they are confident that their relatives will be able to cope with the help of public and private services of sufficiently high quality.

The pattern for Philippine nurses, however, is different. They seem to go abroad and bring their families as soon as they are settled, including parents and siblings. Philippine nurses tend not to return to their native country. There has been no campaign on the part of the Filipino government to encourage return migration—quite the opposite, in fact. The Philippine government has put a greater focus on establishing protective government offices in countries where there are large communities of Filipino migrant workers. The emphasis is servicing their exported workers in the destination countries rather than encouraging them to return to the Philippines. Current policy focuses primarily on addressing staggering levels of unemployment, improving national revenue, establishing positive trade relations with other countries, and providing a higher standard of living for its citizens.

Whether we conceptualize the issue in terms of brain drain, brain gain, or brain circulation will, in a sense, be determined by each country's different priorities. The benefits generated by remittances, the reduction of unemployment in the source country, and return migration must all be weighed carefully. If the source country's priority is increasing the remittances received, policies will be developed that will encourage migration, perhaps reduce unemployment, but definitely not promote return migration. If on the contrary, the shortage of professionals is the priority and strategies are put in place to attract them back, the amount of remittance funds will necessarily decrease. These three policy directions may compete with each other and lead to conflicting interests within decision-making bodies. The end result of negotiations is likely to be different from country to country and will depend on the national circumstances and the priority policy concern, which may change over time.

Researchers have been increasingly interested in return migration, but the data on returnees—their motivations, characteristics, migration patterns, participation in the local labor market, and potential impact—are extremely limited. It is evident, for example, that if only retirees or emigrants who were unsuccessful in the destination country return, their contribution to the economic development of the source country may be less than optimal. The motivation for the return migration will obviously affect its impact.

There have been a few programs specifically encouraging return migration. They have had some success in Turkey, Thailand, Korea, and Taiwan. These initiatives are often very expensive and raise the question, can we afford them in the long term? In large measure, their success was heavily dependent on external factors, namely, a growing economy in the source country that attracted investment as well as professionals. Some economists and migration experts have even wondered if the few success stories of professional migrants returning home would have occurred under these positive circumstances in any case and without these programs.

The special incentives and facilities offered return migrants may in all likelihood generate a degree of frustration and ill will among those who loyally stayed in employment in the source country and never received any assistance. Very limited evaluation of such programs has been undertaken. The International Organization for Migration has initiated several regional programs to encourage return migration to developing countries. Their strategy has changed over the years. Replacing programs focused on "assisted return," the current initiatives like Migration and Development for Africa encourage mobility of people and resources.[94]

Studying brain circulation, rather than brain drain or gain, may be the future for migration experts. If the discussions remain focused on brain drain, as they have for the last forty years, there is no reasonable expectation that they will generate constructive or effective initiatives. The new focus on brain circulation may well provide some key answers to migration flows that can only be expected to increase in the coming years.

7. The Grass *Could* Be Greener . . .

It is a Monday morning in the year 2010, and a nurse in Malawi, the Philippines, or perhaps even Canada or the United Kingdom consults an Internet site which auctions off a variety of hospital nursing jobs available to the entire international nursing community. Like bargaining for Mexican silver jewelry on eBay, the site announces the going bid for the jobs on offer. If the would-be migrant underbids other nurses and her credentials are adequate, she may be the winner.

This scenario may sound utterly implausible but it is not. If massive nurse migration continues unabated, this may be one of the ways migrant nurses find their jobs. Several US hospitals are already promoting an eBay-like auction of nursing shifts as a measure that will both contain costs and retain nurses.[1]

It would be no surprise if this highly controversial workplace innovation were extended globally, since it is grounded in the very same notions that drive much of today's nurse migration. What allows hospital managers to auction shifts—rather than carefully assess which combination of nurses with what mix of skills and experience is best for a particular unit at a given time—is the belief that a nurse is a nurse is a nurse. This is the notion that has allowed administrators and government planners to replace expert nurses with cheaper novice nurses; to float nurses experienced on one unit and in one field (for example, oncology) to another in which they have no experience (say, pediatrics); to replace nurses with lesser-trained aides; or, conversely, to assign experienced nurses to positions and tasks that do not fully utilize their skills. And it is what allows certain policy makers and health economists to attempt floating nurses from one country to another without making sure they are adequately educated and oriented.

This is, of course, the fundamental dilemma of nurse migration. While offering a wide range of opportunities, it also raises serious human/workers' rights issues, challenges the ability of health systems to deliver needed care, and allows them to neglect long-festering workplace problems. The massive migration we see today challenges some strong vested interests while creating others. International mobility is a blunt instrument, often unpredictable because of the multitude of social forces influencing the net flows at any given time.

Continuing to treat the migration of health care workers as a problem, however, does not help minimize whatever negative consequences may exist. When migration is considered the primary disease, efforts tend to focus on artificially curbing or limiting its size, while neglecting the root causes that determine its existence. Restrictive emigration policies, such as the denial of exit visas or curtailing of access to job information, infringe the rights of individuals to make international moves. They are largely counterproductive and may even increase illegal migration.[2] Most important, such measures ignore the reasons that motivate migration and the real benefits that may be gained. "The more we try to deal with migration simply by clamping down on it with tighter border controls, the more we find that human rights are sacrificed—on the journey, at the border, and inside host countries," says Kofi Annan, secretary-general of the United Nations.[3]

The data clearly show that no matter how attractive the pull factors of the destination country, little migration takes place without substantial push factors driving people away from the source country. The reality is that most nurses would prefer to stay at home.

A Question of Choice

How do we create the conditions that make nurses' professional journeys a choice rather than either an obligation or a forced escape? "Most immigrants are not refugees," says Kofi Annan. "We call them *voluntary* migrants—and some of them truly are. However, many leave their home countries not because they really want to, but because they see no future at home."[4]

Make no mistake, nurses all over the world face dire financial need and live in environments where their personal safety, both inside and outside the workplace, is threatened on a daily basis. Access to technological advances, skill development, and independent practice may remain a dream in resource-limited health systems. Educational programs available abroad are often the only way to quench the thirst for further knowledge and broader horizons. In these cases, migration is seen as nurses' first and last chance to make personal and professional development feasible. Is migration motivated by choice or constraint? Although each nurse must be given the liberty to decide, health care workforce planners need to understand the nuances of this question.

Health services that deliberately turn to international recruitment as a way to meet nursing shortages are also making a choice. The aging nursing workforces in industrialized countries may be reinvigorated by integrating the often younger migrant nurses. Their presence is fundamental to the preparation of the next cohort of teachers, clinical mentors, supervisors, and managers. Countries like the United Kingdom, faced with the retirement of one hundred thousand nurses in the next ten years, see the international recruitment of nurses as a necessary strategy if the health needs of their populations are to be met.

Nurse migration is a reality, one that will not be regulated out of existence. The question, however, is to what extent nurse migration will continue on the scale we see today. How can it be managed so that nurse migrants are not subjected to exploitation and unreasonable hardship? How can health care systems, and the patients who depend on them, be protected from the kind of mass migration that will jeopardize their very existence?

In order to enhance the positive benefits and potential of migration, three major issues need to be considered: duration of absence, lost investments, and numbers of migrants. In the face of the economic disparities between industrialized and developing countries, the likelihood that migration will decrease is almost nil. As long as nursing shortages and demand continue to exist, the only factors that will change the phenomenon in the short term are the security issues that emerge because of global terrorism. For example, what if Middle Eastern societies like Saudi Arabia were to become unattractive to foreign nurses because they are afraid of becoming potential political targets? What if Australian universities were to shut off programs in Indonesia because of concerns about terrorism against their citizens? What if a massive SARS or SARS-like epidemic were to sweep over a region from country to country? These "what ifs" just hint at the complications that can inhibit mass nurse migration in a globalized world.

Lowell and Findlay, however, predict migration will continue to exist and suggest that short-term migration is the best option in an "optimal brain drain" world.[5] The distinction between short-term and long-term migration is repeatedly highlighted, with good reason. The period of time away from the source country determines the actual loss to that health system. If allowed to contribute newly acquired knowledge and skills upon return, the migrant nurse will improve patient services and represent not a loss but a definite gain. This is the theory.

Yet, Martineau and colleagues state that there is no proof that the newly acquired knowledge and skills actually make a significant impact in poorly resourced health systems. Of course, the key term here may be "significant." A nurse who returns to her home country can make a contribution and work effectively even if she does not work in a high-tech environment. She will have gained knowledge, been exposed to the latest scientific research, and acquired advanced clinical assessment skills. This nurse can add value to her health care system if she is offered some challenge and an opportunity to advance. But will these be offered? Will countries that fail to retain nurses strive to woo them back?

The duration of nurse migration touches on the question of lost investment by source countries in the education and training of nurses. Many observers of nurse migration also refer to the loss of income taxes that would have been paid by the migrant professionals if they had stayed home. The issue of reparations is raised periodically but is usually set aside quickly. Given the circuitous nature of career paths, described throughout this book, appropriate reparation or compensation will be difficult to determine. What distinctions should be made between temporary and permanent migration? When does temporary become permanent? What happens if the expected loss becomes a gain with return migration? At what point in a particular nurse's migratory journey would payments be made?

Nurse Clarke from Ghana, whom we met in the previous chapter, was obliged to work as a nurse's aide in the for-profit Green Leaves Nursing Home when she moved from Ghana to the United Kingdom. Once fully registered as a nurse, she moved into public-sector hospital work. If some sort of newly created international agency decides that the first destination country, the United Kingdom in this case, will pay the complete education costs in reparation to the source country, Ghana, should the payments correspond to the education costs of a nurse or a nursing assistant? Who would make the payment—Clarke's first employer or the UK government? What happens when Clarke enters the public service? If the Green Leaves Nursing Home paid the initial reparation costs, will it be partially reimbursed when that nurse leaves after one year? Who receives the payment in Ghana—the Ministry of Education, the Ministry of Health, or both? What payment should be expected from South Africa, which was Nurse Clarke's second destination country? If payments are made, must they be reimbursed when the nurse returns home with newly acquired skills and knowledge? And what about poor Nurse Clarke herself? Will anyone bother to compensate her for a year of lost earnings as a nursing home aide?

It would be too difficult to impose a standard "tax" because, as we have seen, the migration paths of nurses are clearly anything but standard. Creating an effective system that would tally all the losses and benefits within any given case over a period of time would be a daunting project. Although the question of reparation will continue to bear on the final evaluation of nurse migration, other measures need to be considered if compensation is to be parceled out systematically. These include the financial support of nursing education systems in the source countries, provision of decent salaries, and employment of adequate levels of staff. Traditionally, donor funds have focused on specific diseases, for example, the eradication of smallpox or more recently the Global Fund to Fight AIDS, Tuberculosis and Malaria. It is time to create a special international fund that will focus on strengthening health systems and the human workforce that delivers patient services. Such a program would concentrate on capacity building in human resources management, job creation, development of educational infrastructures, and provision of incentives to retain health workers in active practice. At the same time, the IMF and World Bank need to relax the financial restrictions applied in developing countries and allow for increased government investment in health and health professionals.

The duration and extent of migration affect source countries in many ways. Excessive levels of skilled emigration deplete the stock of professionals faster than it can be regenerated.[6] There is no definitive formula that determines what is excessive or indicates the optimal level of emigration from a source country. Since there is great variation from one country to another, one cannot make blanket statements about how many nurses can safely leave a particular country or how many a receiving country should optimally accept. For example, the number of Filipino nurses exported represents a significant percentage and sometimes more than the number of new graduates in a particular year. And yet, for many this is considered a positive nurse migration outcome.

Another challenge is the great variation in the scope of practice and qualifications of nurses. The impact of the migrating generalist staff nurse who leaves her work in a tertiary care hospital in the capital city of a developing country may be very different from that of her compatriot who was the sole nurse anesthetist in a rural district far from other referral hospitals. Absolute migration numbers only provide part of the picture. Relative numbers—the percentage of nurses leaving when compared to the remaining stock—as well as personal details of the nurses involved (age, qualifications, years of experience) are equally important in evaluating whatever impact the migration of a given nurse will have. All of this argues for much more detailed data collection, careful planning, and evaluation of the health care workforce than is currently done almost anywhere in the world.

Treatment of the Nurses

Just as health care systems need to be constantly aware of the problems of their homegrown workforce, they also need to understand the stress of migration. It is imperative that nurse migrants be treated with dignity and not as impersonal, disposable cogs on a global assembly line of caregivers. This goes for destination as well as source countries.

Disoriented in new surroundings, far away from the usual support networks, and perhaps limited by language insecurities, migrant workers are even more vulnerable than their homegrown colleagues to discriminatory practices and bad treatment, including poor working and living conditions. The International Council of Nurses declares that numerous migrant nurses have been "employed under false pretences or misled as to the conditions of work and possible remuneration and benefits" and adds that "internationally recruited nurses may be particularly at risk of exploitation or abuse; the difficulty of verifying the terms of employment being greater due to distance, language barriers, cost, etc."[7] Abuse, exploitation, discrimination, and marginalization are unacceptable behaviors. There is no excuse for this kind of widespread psychological violence. It frequently leads to tremendous pain and suffering. Treating nurses fairly and with respect is the fundamental framework necessary for nurse migration to be a positive experience. The fact that migration is being chosen by far more nurses from far more countries than in the past makes the ethical issues involved in nurse migration a lot more pressing. The media sensationalism often associated with reports of migrant exploitation hide the reality that migrant nurses' experience is frequently an exaggerated form of what many local nurses, particularly those from ethnic minorities, encounter on a daily basis. These problems will not disappear with market competition or voluntary codes of practice. To protect nurses and the patients they in turn protect, concrete steps have to be taken to respect workers' rights and regulate the recruitment process.

Social Costs

The social costs of nurse migration cannot be ignored. They exist whether the migrant is male or female. Given the traditional role women play in community and family life, however, the numerical preponderance of women in nursing means these costs may be very high indeed. The fact that migrant nurses are expected to leave their families and home countries—that they are obligated to move thousands of miles away from home in order to fulfill family duties—raises the issue of choice even more starkly.

The social costs of family separation are far reaching. Obviously, hundreds of thousands of individuals are directly affected. As mentioned in previous chapters, parenting becomes all the more challenging. Mothers may need to give up responsibility for their children's upbringing to single fathers, siblings, or aging parents. Roles are interchanged and direct lines of authority may be confused or sporadic. If the family accompanies the nurse on his or her journey, conflict between traditional societal values and those of the destination country may create tensions within the family.

Society in general, however, also suffers some of the impact of disrupted family structures. Fundamental family values that provide the framework for most societies are sometimes weakened or lost by migration and split families. If and when the parents decide to return to the source country, the children who return with their parents may be faced with conflicting pressures and confusion, having perhaps little exposure or loose ties to the culture, the society, and perhaps the language of their native land. The kind of cultural apprenticeship we all go through is made more difficult by distance. This disconnection may threaten the reintegration of the second generation if the family returns to the home country, or weaken obligations to financially support the extended family if they remain in the destination country.

There is yet one more scenario to consider. What happens when a member of the family migrates and the rest follow, including parents and siblings? International legal instruments uphold family (re)unification as a fundamental human right. Many of the major destination countries establish their immigration policy on this premise. For example, the principle of family reunification is widely accepted in the United States as the centerpiece of its immigration policy.[8] It is quite common to have Filipino nurses emigrate to the United States and, over the years, bring their extended family as well. The social cost may be reduced for the individual, but the source country has lost not one health professional but an entire family. Indeed, if enough families leave enough cities and villages, the entire community structure of a country can change in the process.

Under the threat of migrant nurses leaving the country, and to retain a competitive edge in the global labor market, Ireland recently changed its policy of family reunification to allow spouses of non-EU nurses to work. This contrasts with practices in Australia and Canada, which continue to base their migration policy on skills rather than family ties, and with other countries that have restricted migration because of security concerns.

The Nursing Shortage and Patient Safety

Patient safety, when health needs are met under optimal conditions, is the ultimate goal of all health systems. Yet the phenomenon of nurse migration heightens tensions that emerge when an individual's right to migrate competes with humanitarian concerns safeguarding national populations' equitable access to health care. Recruiting individuals from reduced and sometimes seriously depleted skill pools often compromises a country's capacity to deliver quality and equitable health care.

Over the past several decades, research continues to document the significant influence that the size and mix of nurse staffing exerts in the delivery of quality health services, especially in terms of better patient outcomes. Researchers estimate that nurses' high patient loads may account for twenty thousand unnecessary deaths a year in the United States. Indeed, more than fifty research studies have documented the link between inadequate staffing and adverse patient outcomes and mortality.[9]

The US standard allocation of patients per nurse on a medical or surgical unit tends to be four to one. With each additional patient assigned, the risk of burnout increased by 23 percent and the risk of job dissatisfaction by 15 percent.[10] Linda Aiken observes, "There is a threshold level of staffing below which it is not going to be possible to retain other nurses."[11] The link between nurse workload and patient outcomes is critical.

It is clear that until optimal staffing levels are reached, each supplementary nurse brings an added value and improves the quality of care. Internationally recruited nurses, although often essential to maintain services, will in most cases never represent more than a partial and short-term solution to the nursing shortage in destination countries.

Because migrant nurses inevitably will continue to have a role to play, patient safety must rely on competent regulatory bodies that carefully screen applicants wishing to practice as nurses. Trade and economic forces cannot be allowed to jeopardize the professional standing of nurses by facilitating the employment of unqualified people who do not meet the minimum requirements. Protection of the patient is the issue—and not professional protectionism or protection of the profession.

Thus, a key dimension of patient safety is assuring adequate staffing levels in the source countries once nurse migration takes place. The scale of the emigration and its impact once again become cardinal points, bringing us full circle to the factors driving the global nursing shortage.

That so many already fragile health care systems in the third world are now being depleted of nurses—the only caregivers available to huge numbers of sick patients—is perhaps the most controversial issue involved in nurse migration. Shortages in destination countries are the consequence of some of the very same forces that drive nurses to emigrate. Study after study confirms that despite the chaos they create, workforce issues have for decades not received the political attention they deserve. Every time there is a nursing shortage there is global panic. Suddenly organizations and governments form commissions and councils and hold summits and produce a flurry of papers and lengthy lists of recommendations. While research, think tanks, and working groups usually all agree in principle on what must be done to address the nursing crisis, most of the recommendations remain words on the printed page and are never implemented.

In December 1988 a US presidential task force was convened to investigate the nationwide nurse shortage and developed a list of sixteen recommendations for action and change. In 2001 Anne O'Sullivan, representing the American Nurses Association, spoke to the Senate Governmental Affairs Subcommittee when it was investigating shortages in direct care staffing. She pointed out that if the 1988 recommendations had been implemented, there would have been no need for a 2001 meeting to discuss exactly the same issues. If the recommendations continue to be ignored, she predicted, ongoing shortages and additional futile meetings are inevitable.[12] Industrialized as well as developing countries need to accept their responsibilities in comprehensive human resources planning and put in place effective recruitment and retention strategies.

Increasingly, countries are urged to attain self-sufficiency in their health care workforce and avoid generating adverse consequences for other countries. Nurse migration must be seen in its wider context to avoid well-intentioned but damaging policies. For example, responding to the plight of millions affected by the Asian tsunami disaster at the end of 2004, a call was made in the United Kingdom to freeze all recruitment of nurses from India. That same week, however, the Trained Nurses Association of India publicly announced that 60 percent of trained Indian nurses were unemployed. The ethical dilemma of recruiting from nurse-starved health systems exists and must be addressed. Hoping to solve one set of dilemmas but creating another—exacerbating the unemployment of nurses in developing countries—is not a viable approach. There will always, however, be a need for international exchange, and a certain level of migration is welcome and necessary. In the light of recent developments and the increasing number of developing countries producing nurses for export, perspectives on nurse migration may change in the coming years. For example, St. Vincent increased its nursing student enrollments from thirty-five to one hundred per year. Public funds are being invested with full knowledge that only one-quarter of this cohort will be absorbed by the local health system after graduation in 2006. What will happen to these nurses if the international demand disappears? Looking beyond St. Vincent, what will happen to the families dependent on remittances if their relatives lose their jobs as a result of more restrictive immigration policies and are sent back home?

Minimizing the Negative

Nurse migration, under the right conditions, can be beneficial for many of the reasons outlined above. For nurse migration to promise a better life tomorrow, what do we need to know and do now? What mechanisms should we put in place? What issues will determine better nurse retention, minimize shortages, and benefit both homegrown and migrant nurses?

Data

Throughout this book I have referred to the patchiness and sometimes nonexistence of data necessary for a comprehensive analysis of the present situation and sound human resource planning. Many health policy experts and researchers have long argued that the reliable and relevant data upon which good nursing workforce policy depends are simply unavailable. They have valiantly fought for the resources to produce more and better data. Yet their calls remain essentially unanswered.

> Many studies report difficulties of assessing current migration flows and trends. This is in part attributable to the incomplete recording of necessary data. Where information is documented, it is often inaccurate and inconsistent. There also appears to be little international standardization of documentation, making comparison between countries even more complicated. There is also a lack of profession-specific data in relation to nursing; this problem includes differences in categories and definitions in different countries.[13]

When it comes to nurse migration a distinction needs to be made between data on professional registration resulting in a license to practice, on the one hand, and employment details that focus on nurses' work sites, their hours, function, benefits, and pay, on the other. There is often a lack of comprehensive national databases relevant to the nursing labor market or nurses' employment status. What data are available tend to be "fragmented, inconsistent, incomplete, and not comparable nationally or internationally."[14]

Where nurses' professional registration is systematically recorded (and this is not always the case), there is often no way of knowing whether a particular nurse is employed and, if so, where and in what capacity. In federated countries such as the United States and Australia, nurses may be registered in more than one state. They may therefore be counted more than once in national statistics. In most countries and in some states within countries there is no need to renew registration. Once nurses are registered, there is no way to monitor their careers or even know if they are still nursing.

Where the requirement to renew registration exists, nurses may reregister even though they are not working or are employed in some other field.

To make things more complicated, the term *nurse* has no standard international meaning. The term may refer to unskilled and unregulated personnel as well as to registered nurses, which makes occupation-specific comparisons between countries virtually impossible. In the constitution of the International Council of Nurses (ICN), a *registered nurse* is defined as "a person who has completed a nursing education program and is qualified and authorized in her (his) country to practice as a nurse."[15] As this statement implies, there is no universal definition setting common education and practice standards. There is only an acceptance of a wide range of national definitions. Even within countries, the meaning of *nurse* may vary. For example, North Dakota requires a bachelor's degree as the minimum entry qualification for registered nurses. Other states, however, accept nurses with diplomas and associate degrees on their registers.

The verification of qualifications, which occurs when a nurse intends to exercise her profession in another country, is just that—a measure of intention. The nurse may well be registered and then never migrate. For example, Nurse Jacobs[+] from Jamaica may successfully apply to be registered in the United Kingdom but, because of unforeseen familial obligations, change her mind and decide to stay at home. The UK Nursing and Midwifery Council will, nonetheless, have Nurse Jacobs on their register. Based on the registry data, no one can tell if she is employed in the United Kingdom or even if she has ever set foot on UK soil.

In this case, it is obvious that standardized data collection based on agreed terms is required not only to monitor nurse migration but also to have a clear idea of the national nurse workforce at any given time. As seen in previous chapters, it is as important to record the movement of nurses internally as internationally. Understanding the mobility of nurses within countries—from the public to the private sector, from the urban to the rural areas, from active practice to unemployment or employment outside the health sector—is critical for human resource planning and management. Documenting the deployment of nurses—their distribution and hours of service—will yield a clear picture of the nurse workforce in a given country. It will also answer the key question: Is the nursing shortage myth or reality?

System Approaches

Research, however, has to move beyond statistical representations of the problem or promise of nurse migration and must include the voices and concerns of the migrants themselves. Researchers are bound to have an easier time collecting data from migrant nurses who have had good experiences. Exploitation, abuse, or great unhappiness tends to drive nurses to return home or remain silent. In spite of the misery some encounter, it is still true that most migrant nurses report positive experiences. For example, 90 percent of the six hundred Filipino nurses surveyed by UNISON said they would recommend working in the NHS to a friend. Indeed, the majority of these nurses confirm that they would make the same decision if faced with the identical choices. Again, researchers must remember that many of the abuses migrant nurses endure are similar to, or an extreme form of, those that local nurses experience. These include lack of respect, discrimination, overwork, low pay. To right these wrongs, the whole system needs to be reformed. These problems cannot be considered to be "migration issues" and thus be analyzed in isolation from the broader constellation of problems most nurses contend with today. Tackling them as key problems of health-sector employment may unite local and migrant nurses and bridge the divisions that keep them from effectively challenging the structures and policies from which they all suffer.

Regulation

Much of the abuse associated with nurse migration has been blamed on recruitment agents. In the United States nurse leaders today report an improvement in the behavior of agencies after a wave of abuses reported in the 1980s. Ironically, market competition between recruitment agencies, as well as legal action and bad press, has been credited for this change in conduct. Unfortunately, there has been very little political will to systematically regulate these agencies, a move feared to threaten industrial growth and economic prosperity. The regulation of recruitment agencies must nonetheless be part of the strategy if the exploitation of migrant nurses is to be eliminated.

Employers as well as recruitment agencies have misused vulnerable migrant nurses. The ICN calls for "a regulated recruitment process based on ethical principles that guide informed decision-making and reinforce sound employment policies on the part of governments, employers and nurses, thus supporting fair and cost-effective recruitment and retention practices."[16] The council identifies thirteen principles equally relevant for recruitment within a country as between countries: effective human resources planning and development; credible nursing regulation; access to full employment; freedom of movement; freedom from discrimination; good-faith contracting; equal pay for work of equal value; access to grievance procedures; safe work environment; effective orientation/mentoring/supervision; employment trial periods; freedom of association; and regulation of recruitment. While this is a voluntary code, governments would be well advised to incorporate its principles in their legislation. As there is no proof that voluntary codes make a significant impact on real practices, the force of law is required to make a difference.

Obtaining a license to practice in a foreign country is sometimes an unnecessarily long and expensive process. What is required may not be clearly stated. Adaptation and clinical placements may not be sufficiently monitored to identify and weed out fraudulent programs from the system. Exploitation may occur when migrant nurses are trapped in nursing auxiliary positions waiting for their registration to be processed. Patient safety demands a credible and thorough assessment of qualifications, yet the professional regulatory process needs to be streamlined, transparent, and efficient.

The move toward a global harmonization of education standards has begun timidly and will not be realized for many years to come. So long as national needs and health infrastructures continue to vary, so will the nurses' education and practice standards, functions, and roles. The goal of facilitating the international movement of workers will lead to greater efforts to harmonize education standards, and this will include nursing. What is to be avoided at all cost is focusing on the lowest common denominator and introducing a legislatively imposed rigidity that prevents the advancement of the profession. For example, the length of preregistration nursing education programs may vary from two to four years. The minimum starting age of nursing students may range from fourteen to eighteen years, while the educational institutes may be technical high schools, hospital-based programs, or universities. It is understandable that countries where nurses are expected to have the highest level of preregistration education will not lower their standards to that of a high-school vocational program.

Bilateral and multilateral agreements between governments also play a part in the international recruitment and regulation of nurses. Managed migration—which has already been implemented by China and Cuba with African countries and explored by CARICOM with the United States—has been mentioned as a promising option. This program utilizes government-to-government contracts that set the conditions for short-term employment (usually one to three years) after which the return of the migrant nurses to their source country is guaranteed. Managed migration offers a structure that will facilitate temporary employment abroad and ensure reintegration in the source country's public service without loss of employment and seniority benefits. Easy and complete reintegration would be very attractive to nurses who wish to work abroad for only a short period but have been obliged to resort to permanent migration. One word of caution, however.

Only time and systematically collected data will tell if the temporary nature of managed migration is respected. This initiative could become an easy, back-door entry to permanent migration.

For sustainable brain circulation, a critical mass of migrant nurses must be encouraged to return home. Any losses incurred by source countries from the emigration of their nurses, if not already compensated for by remittances or contacts with the diaspora, could be recuperated by the integration of returnees. The fact remains, however, that return migration is often systematically obstructed. Nurses may not have easy access to information with regard to posted vacancies in their countries of origin. If they had resigned from the source country's health system, they will have lost all acquired benefits and salary increases, and will often be reinstated at the bottom of the career ladder. This limits the usefulness of their newly acquired knowledge and skills as well as their access to decision-making positions. Low starting salaries make employment as a nurse unattractive and devalue their professional experience—in both the source and destination countries. The encouragement of return migration to positions commensurate with nurses' qualifications and skill levels is an important strategy to take advantage of the positive benefits and minimize the negative consequences of nurse migration.

Core Labor Rights and Freedoms

Basic workers' rights provide the legitimate framework for employment in any country and must apply to migrant nurses as well as local staff. Nurses must have full access to their core labor rights, which include freedom of association, freedom from discrimination, the right to a safe work environment, equal pay for work of equal value, and easy access to grievance procedures.

Nurse leaders and migrant nurses frequently remark on the difficulty of obtaining the necessary information to make informed decisions. Some cases of abuse have been dismissed, despite the presence of exploitation, because contracts had been signed and the nurse therefore had seemingly agreed to the poor conditions. National nurses' associations are beginning to produce informative materials orienting nurses to work opportunities abroad—and warning, as much as possible, of potential pitfalls or areas where particular attention needs to be given. For example, the Philippine Nurses Association conducts a series of three orientation seminars for nurses interested in working abroad. The International Department of the Royal College of Nursing provides information on health systems and registration procedures for countries that have been attractive to UK nurses over the years. Some associations are looking at the possibility of credentialing "best-practice" agencies instead of "blacklisting" the abusive ones, as was done in the past.

The ICN predicts that "the quality of work life in many health care facilities needs to be improved before high vacancy and turnover rates significantly decrease."[17] We can predict that nurse migration and career moves will therefore continue. In a recent set of Career Move guidelines, nurses considering a change in employment are encouraged to answer the following questions:

- What are the credentials (legitimacy, reputation, or track record) of the recruitment/employment agency?
- What are the credentials of the employer?
- What are the conditions of employment?
- What is the job description?
- What is the impact of this career move?

The best way to control people, of course, is to keep them in the dark. But the potential perils of exploitation and abuse can be avoided when they are recognized in advance. Once in the destination country, the need for reliable information remains essential. Father Claro Conde, a Filipino Catholic priest now working in the United Kingdom, is regularly bombarded with pleas for help. In January 2003 he received more than fifty calls from health workers. With the help of UNISON and Allen Reilly, a retired nurse who heads a Filipino organization in south London, Father Conde created an action group to "rescue" Filipino nurses from the private sector. They disseminated information to local parishes, and the nurses began contacting them. Although a major departure from the traditional relationship between church and labor, this active network has carried out more than five hundred rescue operations since 2000. Nurses have been relocated from the private sector and found jobs in the National Health Service under better conditions. We are told that "the rescue mission goes about clandestinely arranging interviews for the nurses at NHS hospitals. Reilly has even rented out a safe house for the abused nurses."[18]

Nations are beginning to care for their expatriates, extending their embassy and consulate services to provide employment-related counseling and protection against exploitation. Nurses' associations are also creating branches in foreign countries in order to maintain contact, offer support, and facilitate return migration if desired. The national associations of the Philippines, Guyana, and Korea have already created branches abroad and advocate for their members in the political and labor arena. Some unions in both destination and source countries are negotiating partnerships and even providing dual membership to protect their members and facilitate contact with the labor movement.

Professional associations and unions must create more such mechanisms to reach migrant nurses, ease their access to the information they need, and provide support networks. Complementary services can be provided by special departments within national embassies or consulates overseas. Agencies established by the destination country, the employer, or the employment sector can also provide these services. A combination of specially designed programs can be developed to ensure that the necessary assistance is accessible to those in need and in a timely manner.

Integration Strategies

All nurses entering a new workplace need proper orientation, mentoring, and supervision. Migrant nurses are no different, except that their need is perhaps greatest. Their unfamiliarity with the neighborhood, customs, work methods, health system, medical terminology, interpersonal dynamics, and the patient population puts them at a clear disadvantage unless appropriate orientation mechanisms are accessible. Norma Amsterdam, a nurse educated under the British system in Guyana, South America, and now executive vice-president of the 1199/SEIU League of Registered Nurses in New York, confirms that language, cultural adjustments, and assimilation to the professional role played by nurses in the United States are all daunting challenges for the migrant nurse. Migrant nurses' stories highlight the importance of these informal or formal orientation sessions and how much they facilitate the settling-in process—both on the personal and professional level. It is in everyone's interest to have migrant nurses well oriented in their neighborhood and their workplace. Productivity greatly improves, job satisfaction grows, and retention rates increase—all of which maximize the return on the migration investment for the nurses and their employers. In Ireland, a surgical nurse manager told me, the lack of such programs allowed local suspicions to persist and muted the welcome of Filipino nurses.

International Partnerships

Remittances have a powerful economic potential, especially in low-income countries. They can mobilize essential resources for development programs as well as contribute to the survival and well-being of major segments of the population. Improved money transfers will result from streamlining the process, reducing the minimum amounts required for individual transactions, and lowering the cost. Facilitating the transfer of remittances means that a greater proportion of migrant nurses' savings reach their destination for local use in consumption and investment. Government initiatives offering members of the diaspora an option to invest in public projects—for example, building schools, community health centers, and roads reaching the country's interior—will encourage development. Mechanisms to channel funds to effective development projects and programs will improve the productivity and potential impact of remittances. That is why the Group of Seven, representing the world's largest economies, issued a statement at their meeting in February 2004 urging the reduction in transfer fees as a means to address poverty and spur economic growth worldwide.

Members of the diaspora are also participating in new programs where they return to their home country as volunteers to share information, demonstrate technological advances, and develop skills, thereby steadily building the knowledge base and networking capacity of their fellow citizens. Such arrangements have already been initiated by Belgium in Rwanda and Burundi. There is no doubt that the diaspora of nurses provides countries with a rich pool of human as well as financial resources. Contact between the home country and the transnational communities will improve the transfer of information, technology, and funds. These exchanges will in turn encourage productive partnerships between commercial, academic, and service networks in source and destination countries, thus reducing existing economic and developmental gaps. Expatriates continue to need professional networks as well as links with the governments of their native countries. Partnerships have been shown to be very effective, constructive, and supportive of sustainable development.

Recruitment and Retention

According to the International Organization for Migration, "many field studies demonstrate that most people do not wish to immigrate to a foreign country, and that given the choice, many migrants would much prefer to be 'circular' rather than permanent migrants. After all, remaining in one's country of birth is the norm and migration to settle elsewhere the exception."[19] In the history of global migration, most people move because they have reached the end of the options available at home. Any sign that their conditions will improve delays or eliminates the need to migrate. We have seen the case of the Fijian nurses. When the government announced that it would soon evaluate public-sector jobs and thus reclassify nurses and improve their working conditions, the number of Fijian nurses leaving the country dramatically declined. The prospect of better pay and working conditions in the near term convinced nurses to stay at home.

Examples like this demonstrate why the link between nurse migration and nursing shortage is so obvious. If there was no nurse shortage in destination countries, there would be no significant international demand and the most powerful of the current pull factors would disappear. If there were no nurse shortage in source countries, it would mean that the push factors have been addressed. The number of nurses interested in opportunities abroad would decrease to a negligible level.

In the final analysis, nurse shortage stems from an imbalance in the supply and demand for nurses. Nurse supply includes two dimensions that are intrinsically connected: recruitment and retention. To ease a shortage it is critical to bring new recruits into the field or a particular job. These new recruits will not, however, make a difference over the long term unless health care institutions can retain them. Despite this fundamental interdependence, retention has proven to be far more difficult than recruitment.

International recruitment campaigns have been undertaken by employers to deal with the problem of decreasing supply and increasing demand. Even when they are successful, however, they give employers and national health services a false sense of security. Without adequate retention strategies, newly employed nurses seem to leave environments in which poor working conditions prevail almost as quickly as they enter. Sometimes they leave the profession entirely, creating a revolving door in and out of hospitals or nursing. Thus the focus on the recruitment campaign can, in itself, delay effective measures that would improve long-term retention and human resource planning.[20]

If the problem of nurse retention were addressed properly and solved, nurse recruitment would immediately improve and nurse migration would no longer be an issue. Which is why Suzanne Gordon has argued that the common phrase "recruitment and retention" should be reversed and the formulation that more accurately describes the dynamic should be "retention and recruitment."[21] The interrelationship that governs retention and recruitment on the local level applies internationally as well. It is not migration that must be curbed but the need to migrate. If that were to happen, levels of nurse migration would diminish to an optimal level. Then perhaps we could finally focus on how to facilitate brain exchange and brain circulation rather than worry about brain drain and nurse shortage.

Pay and Working Conditions

To retain nurses, workforce issues must be high on the political and management agenda. The rationale is quite straightforward. All advances in the delivery of health care depend on having qualified staff who can deliver needed services to patients. Given how many international reports have rec-ognized the importance of staff and their working conditions, it is a wonder that no comprehensive attempts have been made to rectify the situation. The World Health Organization, the International Labour Organization, the United Nations Development Programme, and even the World Bank all agree that workforce issues have been neglected for too long. Judith Oulton, the ICN chief executive officer, has argued that "health care reform has eroded infrastructures worldwide. Salaries, access to continuing education, everything has suffered." Her concern is that policy makers are not being creative enough to effectively address the shortage.

One first step to assure greater retention of nurses will be to pay nurses better. Not just by increasing their salaries but by correcting the injustice of traditional wage disparities between salaries of nurses and those of other service-sector and professional workers. In Canada, Switzerland, and a number of other countries, nurses have long struggled for pay equity. They ask for equal pay for work of equal value, which, to them, is hardly just a slogan. For more than a decade, nurses have initiated legal challenges to re-dress pay inequities between nurses and other public-sector workers and be-tween nurses and those who do comparable work. While in some cases the nurses have been successful, in at least one case the judge contended that the additional salary disbursement (while justified) would bankrupt the em-ployer and could therefore not be imposed. This kind of double standard ul-timately does a disservice to the public. If governments and health care administrators are to protect their patients, the reality is that they can no longer afford *not* to pay.

Pay equity for nurses, however, will most probably never be achieved through collective bargaining. When salary increases are negotiated, subse-quent pay rises are given to other occupational groups, which thus reinstates the unfair relativities. Other mechanisms, therefore, need to be found to im-pose a major revision of national and institutional pay scales that will truly eliminate the discriminatory gap between nurses' competency levels and pay. Professional unions, such as the New Zealand Nurses Organisation, are undertaking pay equity campaigns to address exactly this issue.

The discriminatory *wage compression* that nurses have suffered for decades has also had serious consequences and must be eliminated. "Most of the wage growth for nurses occurs early in their careers and tapers off with time. The potential for increased earning decreases over time. Conse-quently, as individuals gain seniority, their wages compare less favorably with professionals in comparable jobs, providing a motive for transfer to other careers."[22] The fact is, unlike other professions, there is very little re-ward for professional longevity in nursing. The health care glass ceiling means that nurses are pushed away from the bedside or other clinical areas because they simply do not receive the raises that are common in other fields, and which reward expertise and experience acquired on the job. If nurses are to be encouraged to stay at the bedside and in the profession, pay systems must reflect the added value of their experience, clinical judgment, and in-depth knowledge.

When it comes to nurses in less-developed countries, the problem of remuneration is even starker and more critical. In this case it is not only governments but donors or funders—like those representing tax-funded international development agencies—who exacerbate the problem. Many development agencies have expressed profound reservations about using their aid money to finance salaries and benefits for health care workers like nurses. Given the severity of the global nursing shortage, it is time to reconsider this policy. These policies, although certainly not the dominant factor in creating nurse shortages in developing nations, are part of a broader dynamic that contributes to them. Thus it is no surprise that dramatic nurse vacancy rates are found side-by-side with cases of nurse unemployment in countries like Tanzania, Kenya, and Zambia—all of which receive development aid. While governments and international aid agencies understand the critical nature of these vacancies, in many cases no recruitment effort is being made because "there is no money" to pay for more staff on the payroll or project budget. How do we explain to the people of Grenada that twenty-seven nurse graduates in 2004 found themselves without a job, unable to be absorbed by a financially strapped public health system struggling to cope with the shortage of nurses? How can we explain that Zambia intends to extend the retirement age by ten years to cope with the nursing shortage, while the previous year's nurse graduates are turned away?

It is simply unethical to perpetuate the waste of valuable local nursing skills in health systems crippled by lack of staff. It is time to reconsider development aid policies that could support local nursing staff. There is hope. The 2004 World Health Assembly resolution on international migration calls for the creation of international development partnerships to share management and financial responsibilities for the provision of health care services. These new partnerships would provide the opportunity for innovative approaches to human resource sustainability, including training, recruitment, management, and, in particular, retention strategies. The UK Department for International Development has initiated such a program in Malawi.

According to Peter Heller of the International Monetary Fund, the only viable route for fiscal expansion of domestic revenue (increasing the government budget) for most developing countries is via external grants or con-cessionary loans. He warns that this external money may appreciate the value of local currency which would have a negative effect on the balance of trade. A recent meeting of health stakeholders—titled Overcoming the Crisis—concluded that "while health human resources may be finally gain-ing recognition by the health community, it has barely emerged on the radar screen of economic policymakers."[23] International aid agencies are well aware of the critical nursing shortage and its debilitating effect on popula-tions worldwide. Arguments are being made for the external funding of health worker salaries in exceptional circumstances. Yet, a convincing case for exceptionalism with regard to health human resources seems not to have been made. There is a demand for clarity on "what is exceptional, why [the] exceptional [classification] is necessary, and what will be the implications of urgent exceptional action on the sustainability of long-term efforts."[24] While the discussion continues, development advocates, like Emily Sikazwe of Zambia, remind us that "people are dying and we need to face the moral challenge of making excuses for not doing enough."[25]

Acceptable working conditions need to be introduced at all levels of the health service. Research substantiates the value of adequate staffing levels with high ratios of registered nurses on the nursing team. Significantly bet-ter outcomes for patients and higher job satisfaction for the nurses are in-deed possible. Laws imposing minimum nurse/patient ratios have been introduced in Victoria, Australia, and in California. Soon afterward, five thousand unemployed nurses in Victoria applied to return to work and fill vacant posts in the health services. Working conditions and staffing levels are important. When nurses believe that their work environment allows them to deliver quality care, they are prepared to return to active practice.

Because nursing is predominantly female, employers must also initiate family-friendly employment practices and policies to a far greater degree. During the nursing shortage of the 1980s, employers in the United States drew nurses back into the workforce with better shift options, on-site or near-site child-care centers, and other family-friendly policies. These initia-tives, as well as significant increases in pay, helped alleviate the nursing shortage. The provision of child care and even parent care is often promised but rarely made available. Delivering a twenty-four-hour service makes shift work an inevitable part of clinical nursing. Yet scheduling can be made flexible enough to accommodate family needs. One creative and welcome initiative—the Baylor Plan, developed by the National Institutes of Health in the United States—offered higher rates of pay to nurses working perma-nent weekend shifts. This relieved other nurses from having to work week-ends and rewarded the nurses who did these unpopular shifts. Although the nurses were very happy with the initiative, a number of employers curtailed the program because of the cost. In response, many nurses went on strike to have them reinstated, but with little success. There are solutions—some of them have price tags. But the question for planners and policy makers is this: Is the cost of inaction higher in the long run if nurses are not available to take care of patients?

The elimination of workplace hazards, including violence, must also be addressed and considered a responsibility of employers. Nurses cannot be expected to voluntarily put their lives at risk when they care for patients. Nor should they risk becoming patients themselves as they deliver care. In health care systems strapped for resources, exposing nurses to workplace hazards that make them as sick as their patients is hardly a wise policy option. Yet we see repeatedly that basic protective equipment is unavailable and that personnel policies often neglect pervasive psychological abuse in health-sector workplaces. Until the work environment is made safe, nurses who have a choice will go elsewhere or leave health care altogether.

Furthermore, the same circumstances that make nursing unattractive tarnish the image of the profession for potential new recruits. Measures that increase pay and improve working conditions will automatically enhance nursing's image as a profession and a career. These positive initiatives will make the investment in nurse recruitment pay off in the long term. Because the public often does not have a clear idea of nursing's critical importance in health care, or of the profession's progress and evolution over the past twenty to thirty years, image campaigns are necessary if new recruits are to enter nursing. The professional advances and varied career opportunities, including nursing entrepreneurship ventures, need to be publicized and disseminated to the public and to secondary school leavers who are exploring options for the future. But without significant changes in the workplace, will new recruits stay in active practice long enough to make a difference?

Education

If school leavers decide to enter nursing education programs, sufficient student places must be available to ensure the needed supply of new graduates. These positions may be fully financed or partially subsidized with public monies as a recruitment incentive. In addition, financial support to students should be provided through easily accessible student loans at favorable rates. Finally, governments may decide to introduce bonding systems to guarantee a good return on their investment. Under these programs, new graduates who have benefited from subsidized education can repay their debt either by working for a set number of years or by a cash payment.

Linking the brain drain with reparation costs is misleading. It implies that if a "brain drain tax" is introduced, the problem would be solved. This is clearly not the case. Pumping money into a system does not guarantee the immediate availability of the needed human resources. Nor does it prevent graduates from leaving the country or the profession soon after graduation. The argument supporting reparation implies that if the cost of education and training were somehow recuperated, then the continuing departure of dissatisfied nurses from developing countries would be acceptable. Over the past forty years, many health care experts have argued and documented that reparations do not work, and many now steer clear of any attempt to devise a reparation system. Lowell and Findlay sum up the situation: "A darling of the 1970s, reparation for the direct loss through a 'brain drain tax' has long since been abandoned."[26] This, however, does not exclude the possibility of using development aid to finance educational programs and strengthening the teaching capacity of developing countries, currently being discussed between Canada and CARICOM.

Adequate levels of faculty staff are critical. There has already been a gross reduction of nurse educators (some through migration), and a significant number of aging faculty members will retire in the coming ten to fifteen years. Strategies to increase the number of nurse educators are urgently needed. Ironically, to address the shortage of clinical nurses, some countries have increased the salary of staff nurses, but they neglected raises for nurse educators. In these cases, many nurse educators have abandoned educational institutions and returned to clinical practice. Taking from Paul to pay Peter will not solve the basic problems facing health systems worldwide. Comprehensive strategies must look at all the interdependent parts of the system.

The development of educational programs tailored for nurses who have left active practice also facilitates the return of nurses to the labor market. In Victoria, Australia, staffing ratios and the promise of manageable workloads attracted nurses back into patient care. In many cases, this return was feasible because government offered easily accessible refresher courses. Since nursing is a largely female profession, planners must acknowledge that many nurses will continue to take career breaks when bringing up children. Refresher courses could be very helpful in reaching the pool of unemployed nurses in each country. Assistance in finding employment once the program is finished may also facilitate reentry into the labor market. Producing more nurses, however, is not an answer in itself. Unless investments are made to improve the working conditions and quality of life of nurses in both industrialized and developing countries, nurses will continue to emigrate or abandon the profession.

Professional Autonomy

Nurses often face the dilemma of being held accountable for patient care but being denied the authority to make decisions and exercise their professional autonomy. Health care facilities that value nurses' clinical judgment, encourage their participation in decision making, and grant them autonomy in exercising their profession have better patient outcomes. They also have higher retention rates, lower turnover rates, and even waiting lists of nurses seeking employment. This has been repeatedly documented in the famous Magnet Hospital studies undertaken since the 1980s and confirmed by the American Nurses Credentialing Center—a magnet nursing services accreditation program that is no longer exclusively active in the United States but is going international. Professional autonomy continues to be very dear to nurses, and health employers, colleagues, and patients reap the benefits when it is exercised. Autonomy is a key characteristic of the workplaces that retain nurses in active practice.

Sustainable Health Care Systems

Colorful and vivid images are used to describe international nurse migration. Countries searching for nurses are all "fishing in the same pond," a global labor market. Nurses are on a global "treasure hunt" for a better life, or on a "carousel," in which they "change horses" along the way, all the while hoping to snatch the "golden ring" of a higher standard of living. And finally, health systems are "leaky kettles"—administrators seen to be continually pouring in more and more human resources to maintain services but neglecting to plug the holes that cause the drain.

The reality is that nurses worldwide are essential care providers acting within a complex socioeconomic environment, each of them contributing a unique set of aptitudes, skills, and goals.

Nurse migration may be fraught with serious ethical issues and burdened by the double standards often applied by parties harboring vested interests. Unless new and significant measures are introduced, the nursing crisis and international nurse migration will continue to intensify. The negative as well as positive impacts of that migration will increase. Financial aid to developing countries with depleted nurse workforces is needed to specifically target human resource issues. This may be necessary until a comprehensive and strategic approach to the nurse shortage is implemented and nurses, colleagues, and patients in the developing world experience its positive effects.

Countries with far more resources can profitably lead the way in pioneering durable retention and recruitment strategies. It is an illusion to think that the nursing crisis exists only in the poorer countries. Industrialized countries have ignored the signs that their nurse workforce was suffering. Whether the nursing shortage is myth or reality, one thing is certain—there is a significant pool of nurses who are unwilling to work for the pay and working conditions on offer. And yet, we find the modern paradox—nurses willing to work but refused employment by national health systems unable to absorb them, not for lack of need but for lack of funds. Proper human resource management is long overdue. The emphasis must be placed squarely on this fundamental issue. We must reduce the need to migrate rather than artificially curb the flows, in both industrialized and developing countries.

It comes as no surprise that the pay and working conditions of nurses lie at the crux of the problem. Yet until it becomes obvious that a sustainable and stable nurse workforce is in the interest of policy makers and the public alike, the international global shortage and aggressive recruitment will never end. Self-preservation is one of the most powerful change agents—all other arguments pale in comparison. It is to the benefit of all those who will need nursing care to fight for better working conditions, pay, and authority for nurses.

Nurse migration is pushed, pulled, and shaped by a constellation of social forces and determined by a series of choices made by a multitude of stakeholders. Under the right conditions, and when the final decision to emigrate is a truly voluntary choice, the experience can be wondrous and positive for all. In our globalized world, what all countries need to create is the economic and social framework that will resolve the discrepancies and paradoxes of nurse migration. Only then can migration be part of a sustainable global health care economy that benefits individual nurses, their patients, and the health care institutions in which they work.

Acronyms and Abbreviations

AIDS	acquired immunodeficiency syndrome
ANA	American Nurses Association
APEC	Asia Pacific Economic Cooperation
BBC	British Broadcasting Company
BTA	bilateral trade agreements
CARICOM	Caribbean Community
CGFNS	Commission on Graduates of Foreign Nursing Schools
CNA	Canadian Nurses Association
CRNE	Canadian Registered Nurse Examination
DENOSA	Democratic Nursing Organisation of South Africa
DOH	Department of Health (England)
EEA	European Economic Area
ESB	English-speaking background
EU	European Union
FIU	Florida International University
GATS	General Agreement on Trade in Services
GATT	General Agreement on Tariffs and Trade
GDP	gross domestic product
HANYS	Healthcare Association of New York State
HCA	Hospital Corporation of America
HIV	human immunodeficiency virus
HMO	health maintenance organization
ICN	International Council of Nurses
ILO	International Labour Office
ILO	International Labour Organization
IMF	International Monetary Fund
IOM	International Organization for Migration

IRN	internationally recruited nurse
ITA	international trade agreements
ITO	International Trade Organization
MERCOSUR	Southern Common Market Agreement
MRA	mutual recognition agreement
MTA	multilateral trade agreements
NAFTA	North American Free Trade Agreement
NCLEX-RN	licensing exam for nurses administered by the NCSBN
NCSBN	National Council of State Boards of Nursing of the United States
NESB	non-English-speaking background
NGO	nongovernmental organization
NHS	National Health Service
NMC	Nursing and Midwifery Council
NYSNA	New York State Nurses Association
OECD	Organisation for Economic Co-operation and Development
PSI	Public Services International
PTSD	posttraumatic stress disorders
RCN	Royal College of Nursing
RTA	regional trade agreements
SADC	Southern African Development Community
SARS	severe acute respiratory syndrome
TN	Trade NAFTA
UNCTAD	United Nations Conference on Trade and Development
UNISON	public-sector trade union in the United Kingdom
WHO	World Health Organization
WMA	World Medical Association
WTO	World Trade Organization

Notes

Introduction

1. OECD 2002b.
2. Sison 2002.
3. Stilwell et al. 2003.
4. Artigot 2003.
5. Buchan et al. 2003.
6. Buchan and Sochalski 2004.
7. *AJN* 2002.
8. *ANJ* 2002, 13.
9. Chanda 2002. (In this book I use the US system of numeration, where one billion is 1,000 millions (1,000,000,000) and one trillion is 1,000 billions.)

1. Welcome to Globalization

1. Taylor 2003.
2. IOM 2003a.
3. IOM 2003a.
4. IOM 2003b.
5. Stalker 2000.
6. Martineau, Decker, and Bundred 2002.
7. Buchan and Sochalski 2004.
8. Stilwell et al. 2003.
9. Zachary 2001.
10. Martineau, Decker, and Bundred 2002.
11. Kingma 2001a.
12. Opiniano 2002b.
13. Martineau, Decker, and Bundred 2002.
14. IOM 2003a.
15. Sochalski, Ross, and Polsky 2003, 5.
16. Vujicic et al. 2004.

17. OECD 2002b.
18. Martineau, Decker, and Bundred 2002.
19. Mejia 2004.
20. Padarath et al. 2003.
21. Choy 2003, 102.
22. Galvez Tan 2003, p9.
23. Martineau, Decker, and Bundred 2002.
24. Brown 1997.
25. http://www.netcare.co.za/default.asp?currentpage=basemodule&id=1.
26. Buchan and O'May 1999.
27. Padarath et al. 2003.
28. Padarath et al. 2003.
29. www.cia.gov/cia/publications/factbook/geos/rp.html.
30. Ma. Teresa Soriano of the Institute for Labor Studies, Manila. Presentation at the OECD/WB/IOM Seminar on Trade and Migration, Geneva, 2003.
31. Choy 2003, 15.
32. Choy 2003, 1–2.
33. Choy 2003, 43.
34. Choy 2003, 45.
35. Choy 2003, 73.
36. Choy 2003, 111.
37. Overland 2005.
38. Choy 2003, 19.
39. Ruth Padilla, president of Philippine Nurses Association, presentation at the ICN Workforce Forum, Bangkok, 2004.
40. Choy 2003.
41. Choy 2003.
42. Cruz 2004, 62.
43. Armstrong 2003.
44. Allan and Larsen 2003.
45. Hanhel 1999, 52.
46. Colgan 2002 as quoted by GATSwatch (www.gatswatch.org).
47. Liese, Blanchet, and Dussault 2003, 9.
48. Liese, Blanchet, and Dussault 2003.
49. Liese, Blanchet, and Dussault 2003, 8.
50. WHO 2003, 110.
51. Huddart and Picazo 2003.
52. Liese, Blanchet, and Dussault 2003.
53. www.doh.gov.za/docs/pr/2004/pr0128.html.
54. Petros 2003.
55. Finlayson et al. 2002b, 544.
56. Liese, Blanchet, and Dussault 2003.
57. Kingma 2001b.
58. Aiken 2001, 6.
59. Liese, Blanchet, and Dussault 2003.
60. Adams and Al-Gasseer 2001.
61. O'Sullivan 2001.

62. Baumann et al. 2004, 12.
63. www.cia.gov/cia/publications/factbook/geos/us.html.
64. Aiken 2001.
65. Aiken et al. 2002.
66. Aiken 2001, 10.
67. Baumann et al. 2004.
68. Sochalski 2002.
69. Baumann et al. 2004.
70. JCAHO 2002, 10.
71. ANA 2001.
72. Aiken 2001.
73. Hopkins 2001.
74. RCN 2003, 1.
75. ICN 2003c.
76. Buerhaus, Staiger, and Auerbach 2003.
77. CNA 2002a.
78. O'Sullivan 2001.
79. Abelson 2002, 1–3.
80. Gonzales 2003.
81. Fletcher 2002.
82. CNA 2002b.
83. Dinsdale 2003.
84. Crouch 2003, 23.
85. Di Martino 2002.
86. Di Martino 2002.
87. Aiken et al. 2001.
88. Gordon 2005.
89. Mason 2002b, 7.
90. Fischman 2002.
91. *NT* 2001, 4.
92. Baumann et al. 2001, i.
93. Kingma 2003.
94. BBC News 1999.
95. Anon. 2004, 8.
96. Gage, Pope, and Lake 2002; Brown and Connell 2004.
97. Cowin and Jacobsson 2003.
98. Mann 1987.
99. Minton 1998.
100. O'Sullivan 2001.
101. O'Dowd 2002.
102. Editor 2003a, 5.
103. Finlayson et al. 2002a.
104. RCN 2003.
105. Finlayson et al. 2002a.
106. Kai Tiaki Nursing 2002.
107. INO 2003.
108. Adams and Al-Gasseer 2001.

109. JCAHO 2002, 10.
110. ICN 2001b.
111. Condon 2004.
112. OECD 2004a.
113. Aiken et al. 2001, 48–49.
114. Buchan 2002b, 752.
115. S. Lewis 2002, 1362.
116. Hurst and Siciliani 2003.
117. OECD 2002b.
118. Padarath et al. 2003, 18.
119. ILO 2005.
120. Huddart and Picazo 2003.
121. Liese, Blanchet, and Dussault 2003.
122. Scottish Executive 2004.
123. Nolen 2004.
124. IRIN 2004.
125. UNAIDS/WHO 2004.
126. B. Stilwell, interview.
127. Anon. 2002.
128. Kisken 2004.
129. Janofsky 2002.
130. ICN 2000a.
131. Buchan 2002a.
132. OECD 2002b.

2. The Human Face of Nurse Migration

1. See www.unison.org.uk/equalpay/issues.asp.
2. Padarath et al. 2003.
3. ILO 1998.
4. ICN 2000b.
5. Commonwealth Secretariat 2001, 24.
6. Awases et al. 2004.
7. Chappell and Di Martino 2000.
8. Di Martino 2002.
9. Pinder 2002.
10. ILO 1998.
11. Mejia 2004.
12. Brecher 2003, 2.
13. Kingma 1999.
14. Omeri and Atkins 2002.
15. Omeri and Atkins 2002.
16. Spencer 2003/4, 14.
17. Hawthorne 2001.
18. Hawthorne 2001.
19. Hawthorne 2001, 225.
20. Allan and Larsen 2003, 102.

21. Mason 2002a.
22. E. Lewis 2002, 13.
23. Ball and Pike 2004.
24. Ryan 2003.
25. RCN 2002.
26. Sarpong 2002.
27. *NT* 2003b, 4.
28. Santiago 2003, 1.
29. Payne 2003.
30. *NT* 2003a.

3. Mini-Business, Big Business

1. Salt 2001, 88–89.
2. Gamble 2002, 176.
3. UN ECLAC 2003.
4. Salt 2001.
5. www.cgfns.org.
6. Xu 2003, 273.
7. Xu 2003, 270.
8. Shevel 2003, 1.
9. Bach 2003.
10. Choy 2003, 111–12.
11. AACN 2003, 4.
12. AACN 2003, 4.
13. www.netcare.co.za/Default_site.asp?WCI=pgPress&pressid=57.
14. Brecher 2003, 2.
15. Brecher 2003.
16. Costello 2002.
17. AHA 2002.
18. Letter from the management I.Q.MAN (International Quality Manpower Services, Inc.), the land-based counterpart of one of the largest suppliers of Filipino seafarers, the C.F. Sharpe Group.
19. Stone and Hill 2003.
20. Mulholland 2003.
21. Philip Martin, presentation at the OECD-World Bank-IOM Seminar on Trade and Migration, November 2003.
22. Salt 2001.
23. Gordon and Wroe 2003.
24. AusStats 2003.
25. Maiden 2003.
26. AusStats 2003.
27. Lindsay 2003/4.
28. R. Aitken, personal communication with Suzanne Gordon.
29. La Trobe University 2004.
30. www.cambridge-efl.org/exam/general/bg_cpe.cfm.
31. Jordan 2000.

32. Jordan 2000, 9.
33. ICN 2003b.
34. NCSBN 2004.
35. www.ncsbn.org.
36. Choy 2003.
37. CGFNS 1999.
38. E. Sanders, personal interview.
39. www.cgfns.org/cgfns/programs/ice.html.
40. www.cgfns.org/cgfns/programs/icd.html.
41. CGFNS 1999, 2.
42. B. Nichols, personal communication. The alert was titled "Claim of Visa Assist Program Inc. to be Authorized to Issue Section 343 Certificates to Foreign Health Care Workers."
43. Kenny 2002, 3.
44. Allan and Larsen 2003, 44.
45. Pearce 2003, 16.
46. Mulholland 2002a.
47. Barry et al. 2003, 34.
48. Janofsky 2002.
49. HANYS 2003.
50. Larson 2004.
51. Ginsberg 2004.
52. AHA 2003.
53. NCSBN 2003.
54. www.nzno.org.nz/SITE_Default/SITE_About_Us/Kai_Tiaki/Advertising.asp.
55. http://travelnursing.com.
56. Spencer 2003/4, 15.
57. Choy 2003.
58. Carvajal 2004.
59. Carvajal 2004.
60. P. Wickramasekara, interview.
61. IOM 2003a.
62. S. Lipat, interview.
63. Martin 2003b, 2.
64. Stewart 1998.
65. Choy 2003.
66. ANA 1998.
67. See Salt 2001.
68. Mcgarvie 2004.
69. Taylor 2003.
70. Martineau, Decker, and Bundred 2002, 11.
71. Mcgarvie 2004, 1.
72. Opiniano 2002a, 1.
73. Opiniano 2002a, 1.
74. Allan and Larsen 2003.
75. Omeri and Atkins 2002.
76. NT 2003c.

77. Opiniano 2002b.
78. BBC News 2003, 1.
79. HRW 2000.
80. ICN 1996.
81. Power 2004, 6.
82. OECD 2002b.
83. ICN 2001a, 1.
84. Atencio, Cohen, and Gorenberg 2003; Kosel and Olivio 2002.
85. Bach 2003, 19–20.
86. Bach 2003.
87. UNHCHR 2003.
88. Macan-Markar 2003, 2.

4. Vested Interests, Inconsistencies, Double Standards

1. *Accra Mail* 2001.
2. Abacci Atlas 2004.
3. SouthAfrica.info 2004.
4. Commonwealth Secretariat 2001.
5. Martineau, Decker, and Bundred 2002.
6. Commonwealth Secretariat 2001.
7. Martineau, Decker, and Bundred 2002.
8. Couper and Worley 2003.
9. SouthAfrica.info 2004.
10. Gaither 2000, 2.
11. Department of Health 1999, 11.
12. Anon. 2000, 13.
13. Editor 2000.
14. Buchan, Parkin, and Sochalski 2003.
15. Willetts and Martineau 2004.
16. Mulholland 2004, 1.
17. Mulholland 2004, 1.
18. Buchan and Sochalski 2004, 5.
19. Commonwealth Secretariat 2001.
20. Willetts and Martineau 2004.
21. Bach 2003, 23.
22. Buchan, Parkin, and Sochalski 2003.
23. Bach 2003.
24. Mulholland 2002b, 3.
25. *NT* 2003d, 13.
26. Commonwealth Secretariat 2003.
27. Commonwealth Secretariat 2001, 17.
28. Dugger 2004, 1.
29. SADC 2001.
30. ILO 1992.
31. ICN 1999c.
32. Nelson 2001.

33. Gordon 2005, 128–33.
34. Islam 2003, 1.
35. Islam 2002.
36. Islam 2002.
37. WMA 2003.
38. Commonwealth Secretariat 2004.

5. Trade and Migration

1. PSI 1997, 6.
2. www.wtolorg/english/docs_e/legal_e/26-gts.pdf.
3. Aaronson 2001, 3.
4. Martin 2003c.
5. Adlung and Carzaniga 2002.
6. OECD 2002a.
7. OECD 2004b.
8. WTO 2004b, 1.
9. Aaronson 2001, 1–2.
10. Cutshall 2000.
11. Nielson and Taglioni 2003, 4.
12. Nielson and Taglioni 2003, 5.
13. Mattoo 2003, 3.
14. Chanda 2002.
15. WTO 1995.
16. Bugalama 2004.
17. Milholland 2000.
18. Milholland 2000, 8.
19. Chanda 2002.
20. Chanda 2001.
21. Cutshall 2000, 40.
22. http://www.info-seek.co.uk/results.php?keyword=eye%20surgery.
23. www.csmngt.com/medical2.htm.
24. http://www.dtcuba.com/eng/buscar:reportajes.asp?cod=11.
25. Fawthrop 2004, 2.
26. Chanda 2001, 8–9.
27. UNCTAD 1997b.
28. Chanda 2002.
29. Mattoo 2003, 3.
30. http://docsonline.wto/org.
31. http://docsonline.wto/org.
32. Nielson and Taglioni 2003, 7.
33. Winters et al. 2002.
34. Adlung and Carzaniga 2002, 14.
35. Adlung and Carzaniga 2002.
36. GATSwatch 2004, 1.
37. Lovell 2004, 1.
38. Stiglitz 2002, 4.

39. Woodward et al. 2002, 8.
40. ICN 1999a.
41. www.gatswatch.org/about.html.
42. Chanda 2002, 41.
43. UNCTAD 1997a.
44. WTO 2004a.
45. Cutshall 2000.
46. WTO 1998a, 1.
47. WTO 1998b, 1.
48. Mattoo 2003.
49. Nielson 2003a.
50. Nielson 2003a.
51. Nielson 2003a.
52. Cutshall 2000.
53. Cutshall 2000.
54. Later the name was changed to the European Community (EC) and then the European Union (EU).
55. Cutshall 2000, 15.
56. Personal communication.
57. Harrison and Duffin 2003, 8.
58. *NS* 2003, 9.
59. *NT* 2002, 5.
60. *NS* 2003.
61. ICN 2003a, 1.
62. Alexander and Runciman 2003.
63. Nielson 2003b.
64. Nielson 2003b, 8.
65. Nielson 2003b, 19.
66. Cutshall 2000, 22.
67. Iredale 2003, 9.
68. Iredale 2003, 10.
69. Hawthorne 2001, 221.

6. Brain Drain, Brain Gain, Brain Circulation

1. Woodward et al. 2002.
2. Martineau, Decker, and Bundred 2002.
3. Stilwell et al. 2003.
4. Padarath et al. 2003.
5. OECD 2003.
6. Wayne 2004.
7. Iredale 2001.
8. Connolly 2001.
9. Jourdan 2003.
10. Merckling 2003b.
11. Merckling 2003b.
12. Merckling 2003a.

13. Sison 2002.
14. Iredale 2001, 8.
15. Lowell and Findlay 2002, 4.
16. Wickramasekara 2003.
17. Ghose 2003.
18. Martin 2003a.
19. Liese, Blanchet, and Dussault 2003, 10.
20. OECD 2002b.
21. Padarath et al. 2003.
22. IOM 2003a.
23. Ratha 2003.
24. Andrews 2004, 30.
25. Martineau, Decker, and Bundred 2002.
26. OECD 2002b.
27. Mfula 2003.
28. Cited in Wickramasekara 2003, 8.
29. WHO 2004a, 3.
30. Slavery 2003, 4–5.
31. UN ECLAC 2003, 14–15.
32. Kingma 2001a.
33. Parris 2001, 5.
34. OECD 2002b.
35. Wickramasekara 2003.
36. Lowell and Findlay 2002, 6.
37. Wayne 2004, 30.
38. Wayne 2004, 30.
39. Martineau, Decker, and Bundred 2002, 11.
40. Allan and Larsen 2003, 63.
41. Lowell and Findlay 2002.
42. Lowell and Findlay 2002, 7.
43. Lowell and Findlay 2002.
44. Hawthorne 2001, 226.
45. Trossman 2002.
46. Trossman 2002, 2.
47. Berger 2003, B1.
48. Opiniano 2003.
49. Crampton 2003, 13.
50. US Census Bureau 2000.
51. US HHS/HRSA/BHPR 2002.
52. Moore et al. 2005.
53. UN ECLAC 2003.
54. HANYS 2003.
55. WHO 2004b, 2.
56. Commonwealth Secretariat 2003, 14–15.
57. SADC 2001.
58. Padarath et al. 2003, 21.
59. IOM 2003a, 17, 229.

60. Carvajal 2004.
61. Martineau, Decker, and Bundred 2002.
62. Verbal communication during Expert Meeting on Market Access Issues in Mode 4 and Effective Implementation of Article IV on Increasing the Participation of Developing Countries, Geneva, July 29–31, 2003.
63. IOM 2003a.
64. Lowell and Findlay 2002.
65. Ratha 2003.
66. Lowell and Findlay 2002.
67. Ratha 2003.
68. OECD 2002b.
69. Connell and Brown 2004.
70. Brown 1997.
71. Ratha 2003.
72. Brown 1997.
73. World Bank 2003, 2.
74. Ratha 2003.
75. Lowell and Findlay 2002.
76. Ratha 2003, 161.
77. Kochubka et al. 2002.
78. PNB Trust Banking Group 2004.
79. Ratha 2003.
80. *Times of India* 2000.
81. Lowell and Findlay 2002.
82. University Public Relations 2001.
83. Lowell and Findlay 2002.
84. Padarath et al. 2003.
85. Brown 1997.
86. Hampshire 2003.
87. Penn Nursing 2004.
88. Ghosh 2000, 189–90.
89. King 2000.
90. Martineau, Decker, and Bundred 2002.
91. Martineau, Decker, and Bundred 2002, 10.
92. Stephens 2003, 14.
93. Editor 2003b.
94. Wickramasekara 2003.

7. The Grass *Could* Be Greener . . .

1. Chang 2004.
2. Lowell and Findlay 2002.
3. Annan 2003, 3.
4. Annan 2004, 2.
5. Lowell and Findlay 2002.
6. Lowell and Findlay 2002.
7. ICN 2001a, 5.

8. IOM 2003a.
9. Webber 2000.
10. Aiken et al. 2002.
11. Parish 2003, 5.
12. O'Sullivan 2001.
13. Buchan, Parkin, and Sochalski 2003, 9.
14. Baumann et al. 2004, 4.
15. ICN 2001c.
16. ICN 2001a, 1.
17. ICN 2002, 11.
18. Grzincic 2004, 4.
19. IOM 2003a, 6.
20. ICN 1999b.
21. Gordon, interview.
22. Baumann et al. 2004, 15.
23. Chen 2005 4.
24. Chen 2005, 4–5.
25. Chen 2005, 4.
26. Lowell and Findlay 2002, 18.

References

AACN (American Association of Colleges of Nursing). 2003. "Thousands of Students Turned Away from the Nation's Nursing Schools Despite Sharp Increase in Enrollment." December. http://www.aacn.nche.edu/Media/NewsReleases/enrl03.htm (accessed 7 May 2005).

Aaronson, Susan A. 2001 "From GATT to WTO: The Evolution of an Obscure Agency to One Perceived as Obstructing Democracy." *EH.Net Encyclopedia*, edited by Robert Whaples. August 15. http://www.eh.net/encyclopedia/contents/aaronson.gatt.php (accessed 7 May 2005).

Abacci Atlas. 2004. "The Economy of South Africa." http://www.abacci.com/atlas/economy.asp?countryID=323 (accessed 7 May 2005).

Abelson, Reed. 2002. "Patients Surge and Hospitals Hunt for Beds." http://www.weinsurehealth.com/PatientsSurgeintoHospitals.pdf (accessed 7 May 2005).

Accra Mail. 2001. "Ghana: Bolgatanga Nursing Training Cannot Admit New Students." *Accra Mail* August 23 http://www.africaonline.com/search/search.jsp?a=v&contentid=27502&languageid(accessed 6 November 2003).

Adams, Orvill, and Naeema Al-Gasseer. 2001. "Strengthening Nursing and Midwifery: Process and Future Directions—Summary Document, 1996–2000." Geneva: World Health Organization. http://www.who.int/health-services-delivery/nursing/who_eip_osd_2001.5en/who_eip(accessed 7 May 2005).

Adlung, Rudolph, and Antonia Carzaniga. 2002. "Health Services under the General Agreement on Trade Services." In *Trade in Health Services: global, regional, and country perspectives,* edited by Nick Drager and Cesar Vieira, 13–33. Washington DC: Pan American Health Organization.

AHA (American Hospital Association). 2002. "Tenet Awards $1 Million to Train Latino Nurses in Los Angeles." http://www.hospitalconnect.com/aha/jsp/display.jsp?dcrpath=AHA/NewsStory_Artic(accessed 11 January 2004).

——. 2003. "DHS rule requires new certification for overseas health professionals." http://www.hospitalconnect.com/ahanews/jsp/display.jsp?dcrpath=AHA/NewsStory_A(accessed 7 May 2005).

Aiken, L. H. 2001. "The Hospital Nurse Workforce: Problems and Prospects." Prepared for the Council on the Economic Impact of Health System Change,

University of Pennsylvania. http://www.sihp.brandeis.edu/council/pubs/
hospstruct/council-Dec-14–2001-(accessed 7 May 2005).

Aiken, Linda H., Sean P. Clarke, Douglas M. Sloane, Julie A. Sochalski, Reinhard
Busse, Heather Clarke, Phyllis Giovannetti, Jennifer Hunt, Anne Marie Rafferty, and
Judith Shamian. 2001. "Nurses' Reports on Hospital Care in Five Countries." *Health
Affairs,* May/June, 43–53.

Aiken, Linda H., Sean P. Clarke, Douglas M. Sloane, Julie Sochalski, and Jeffrey H.
Silber. 2002. "Hospital Nurse Staffing and Patient Mortality, Nurse Burnout, and Job
Dissatisfaction." *Journal of the American Medical Association* 288 (16): 1987–93.

AJN (American Journal of Nursing). 2002. "Hospitals in Crisis." *American Journal of
Nursing* 102(7):20.

Alexander, Margaret F., and Phyllis J. Runciman. 2003. *ICN Framework of Competencies
for the Generalist Nurse.* Geneva: International Council of Nurses.

Allan, Helen, and John Aggergaard Larsen. 2003. *"We Need Respect": Experiences of
Internationally Recruited Nurses in the UK.* London: Royal College of Nursing.

ANA (American Nurses Association). 1998. "American and Foreign Nurses Abused
by Massive Visa Fraud." http://nursingworld.org/pressrel/1998/foreign.htm
(accessed 7 May 2005).

——. 2001. "Nurses Say Health and Safety Concerns Play Major Role in Employment
Decisions." September 7. http://nursingworld.org/pressrel/2001/pr0907b.htm
(accessed 7 May 2005).

Andrews, Cathy. 2004. "This Is Why We Are Choosing to Leave the UK and Work
Abroad." *Nursing Standard* 18 (22): 30.

Annan, Kofi. 2003. "Emma Lazarus Lecture on International Flows of Humanity."
November 21. http://www.un.org/News/Press/docs/2003/sgsm9027.doc.htm
(accessed 7 May 2005).

——. 2004. "Address to the European Parliament upon Receipt of the Andrei
Sakharov Prize for Freedom of Thought." January 29. http://europa-eu-un.org/
article.asp?id=3178 (accessed 21 November 2003).

Anonymous. 2000. "South African Nurses Banned from Working in the UK." *Nursing
Update* February/March, 13.

——. 2002. "US Looks Abroad for Nurses." *Australian Nursing Journal* 10 (4): 23.

——. 2004. "National Petition Reaches Parliament." *Kai Tiaki Nursing New Zealand.*
July, 8.

Armstrong, Fiona. 2003. "Finding a Sustainable Solution." *Australian Nursing Journal*
11 (3): 24–26.

Artigot, Florencio. 2003. "Les hôpitaux canadiens battent le rappel des infirmières
québécoises exilées en Suisse." *Le Temps,* October 17. http://www.letemps.ch/
(accessed 15 January 2004).

Atencio, Bonnie, Jayne Cohen, and Bobbye Gorenberg. 2003. "Nurse Retention: Is It
Worth It?" *Nursing Economics* 21:262–68.

AusStats (Australian Bureau of Statistics). 2003. "Full-Fee Paying Overseas Students."
In *Education and Training, Year Book Australia 2003.* http://www.abs.gov.au/
Ausstats/abs@.nsf/0/8ec06f7e98a0a4d7ca256cae000ff0d9?Op (accessed 7 May
2005).

Awases, M., J. Nyoni, A. Gbary, and R. Chatora. 2004. *Migration of Health Professionals
in Six Countries: A Synthesis Report.* Harare: World Health Organization Regional
Office for Africa.

Bach, Stephen. 2003. *International Migration of Health Workers: Labour and Social Issues—A Working Paper.* Geneva: International Labour Office.

Ball, Jane, and Geoff Pike. 2004. *Stepping Stones: Careers of Nurses in 2003.* London: Royal College of Nursing.

Barry, Jean, Louise Sweatman, Lisa Little, and Janet Davies. 2003. "International Nurse Applicants." *Canadian Nurse* 99 (8): 34.

Baumann, Andrea, Jennifer Blythe, Camille Kolotylo, and Jane Underwood. 2004. "The International Nursing Labour Market Report." In *Building the Future: An integrated Strategy for Nursing Human Resources in Canada.* Ottawa: Nursing Sector Study Corporation.

Baumann, Andrea, Linda O'Brien-Pallas, Marjorie Armstrong-Stassen, Jennifer Blythe, René Bourbonnais, Sheila Cameron, Diane Irvine Doran, Michael Kerr, Linda McGillis Hall, Michel Vzina, Michelle Butt, and Leila Ryan. 2001. *Commitment and Care: The Benefits of a Healthy Workplace for Nurses, Their Patients and the System—A Policy Synthesis.* Ottawa: Canadian Health Services Research Foundation.

BBC News. 1999. "Why an NHS Nurse Is Hard to Find." *BBC News,* February 1. http://news.bbc.co.uk/1/hi/health/251376.stm (accessed 7 May 2005).

———. 2003. "UK 'Racist' to Overseas Nurses." *BBC News,* July 21. http://news.bbc.co.uk/1/hi/health/3083729.stm (accessed 7 May 2005).

Berger, Joseph. 2003. "From Philippines, with Scrubs." *New York Times,* November 24, B1.

Brecher, Elinor J. 2003. "Program Gets Foreign-Born Physicians Back into Healthcare Profession." *Miami Herald.* http://allnurses.com/t52622.html (accessed 7 May 2005).

Brown, Dennis A. 1997. "Workforce Losses and Return Migration to the Caribbean." In *Caribbean Circuits—New Directions in the Study of Caribbean Migration,* edited by Patricia R. Pessar, 197–223. New York: Center for Migration Studies of New York.

Brown, Richard, and John Connell. 2004. "The Migration of Doctors and Nurses from South Pacific Island Nations." *Social Science and Medicine* 58:2193–2210.

Buchan, James. 2002a. *International Recruitment of Nurses: United Kingdom Case Study.* London: Royal College of Nursing.

———. 2002b. "Global Nursing Shortages." *British Medical Journal* 324:751–52.

Buchan, James, and F. O'May. 1999. "Globalisation and Healthcare Labour Markets: A Case Study from the United Kingdom." *Human Resources for Health Development Journal* 3 (3): 199–209.

Buchan, James, Tina Parkin, and Julie Sochalski. 2003. *International Nurse Mobility: Trends and Policy Implications.* Geneva: World Health Organization.

Buchan, James, and Julie Sochalski. 2004. "Nurse Migration: Trends and the Policy Context." Unpublished.

Buerhaus, Peter I., Douglas O. Staiger, and David I. Auerbach. 2003. "Is the Current Shortage of Hospital Nurses Ending?" *Health Affairs* 22 (6): 191–98.

Bugalama, Habby R. L. 2004. "Urgent Request For Clinical Advice." Personal communication.

Carvajal, Doreen. 2004. "Untapped Potential of the Money Lifeline." *International Herald Tribune,* February 21–22, 1, 13.

CGFNS (Commission on Graduates of Foreign Nursing Schools). 1999. "Alert: Important Information." Philadelphia: CGFNS. http://www.cgfns.org/cgfns/newsandevents/importantinfo.html (accessed 24 February 2004).

Chanda, Rupa. 2001. *Trade in Health Services.* CMH Working Paper Series, no. WG4:5. Geneva: World Health Organization, Commission on Macroeconomics and Health.
———. 2002. "Trade in Health Services." In *Trade in Health Services: Global, Regional, and Country Perspectives,* edited by Nick Drager and Cesar Vieira, 35–44. Washington, DC: Pan American Health Organization.
Chang, Alicia. 2004. "Hospitals Try Online Staffing." *Chicago Tribune,* 13 January. http://www.chicagotribune.com/classified/jobs/chi-0401130322jan13,0,6515487 .stor (accessed 5 February 2004).
Chappell, Duncan, and Vittorio Di Martino. 2000. *Violence at Work.* Geneva: International Labour Office.
Chen, Lincoln. 2005. "Triple C's in Oslo: Consultation, Consensus, and Call-for-Action." Report of the meeting Overcoming the Crisis: Taking Forward the Abuja Action Agenda. Unpublished.
Choy, Catherine Ceniza. 2003. *Empire of Care: Nursing and Migration in Filipino American History.* Durham: Duke University Press.
CNA (Canadian Nurses Association). 2002a. "CNA Aims to Renew Nursing Workforce." *Canadian Nurse* 98 (9): 28.
———. 2002b. *Planning for the Future: Nursing Human Resource Projections.* Ottawa: Canadian Nurses Association.
Colgan, Ann-Louise. 2002. "Hazardous to Health: The World Bank and IMF in Africa." *Africa Action,* April 18.
Commonwealth Secretariat. 2001. *Migration of Health Workers from Commonwealth Countries: Experiences and Recommendations for Action.* London: Commonwealth Secretariat.
———. 2003. *Commonwealth Code of Practice for the International Recruitment of Health Workers.* London: Commonwealth Secretariat.
———. 2004. "Working Group On Teacher Recruitment." *Commonwealth Secretariat News,* March 4. http://www.thecommonwealth.org/Templates/System/ LatestNews.asp?NodeID=36726 (accessed 7 May 2005).
Condon, Deborah. 2004. "Talent Pool Lies Dormant." *World of Irish Nursing,* January, 16–17.
Connell, John, and Richard P. C. Brown. 2004. "The Remittances of Migrant Tongan and Samoan Nurses from Australia." *Human Resources for Health* 2 (2): 1–21. http://www.human-resources-health.com/content/2/1/2 (accessed 7 May 2005).
Connolly, Niamh. 2001. "Health Board Looks to China for Nurses." *Sunday Business Post* (Ireland), September 9. http://archives.tcm.ie/businesspost/2001/09/ 09/story305334.asp (accessed 5 January 2004).
Costello, Mary Ann. 2002. "CA Program Aids Foreign-Trained Professionals." http://www.hospitalconnect.com/jsp/article.jsp?dcrpath=AHA/NewsStory _Article/d(accessed 11 January 2004).
Couper, Ian, and Paul Worley. 2003. "The Ethics of International Recruitment." *International Electronic Journal of Rural and Remote Health Research, Education, Practice and Policy.* http://news.bbc.co.uk/1/hi/health/3083729.stm (accessed 1 March 2004).
Cowin, Leanne, and Denise Jacobsson. 2003. "The Nursing Shortage: Part Way Down the Slippery Slope." *Collegian* 10 (3): 31–35.
Crampton, Joy. 2003. "Foreign Nurses Are Highly Valued Members of the NHS." *Nursing Times* 99 (18): 13.
Crouch, David. 2003. "As If by Magic." *Nursing Times* 99 (2): 21–23.

Cruz, Booma. 2004. "It's Not Brain Drain, It's Hemorrhage: The Shortage of Nurses in the U.S. and the U.K. Has Triggered an Exodus. Now the Philippines' Health Care System Is on the Verge of Collapse." *Filipinas Magazine* 13 (145): 60–63, 69.

Cutshall, Pat. 2000. *Understanding Cross Border Professional Regulation: What Nurses and Other Professionals Need to Know.* Geneva: International Council of Nurses.

Department of Health. 1999. *Guidance on International Nursing Recruitment.* London: Department of Health.

Di Martino, Vittorio. 2002. *Workplace Violence in the Health Sector: Country Case Studies—Synthesis Report.* Geneva: International Labour Office.

Dinsdale, Paul. 2003. "Most Wards Function with Inadequate Staffing Levels." *Nursing Standard* 17 (33): 5.

Dugger, Celia W. 2004. "An Exodus of African Nurses Puts Infants and the Ill in Peril." *New York Times,* July 12, A-1.

Editor. 2000. "Nursing Times Provide Key Points in International Recruitment of Nurses." *Nursing Update,* May, 5.

——. 2003a. "Figures Show Nursing Crisis Worse." *Australian Nursing Journal* 11 (1): 5.

——. 2003b. "Jamaica: Brain Gain." *Economist,* October 9.

Fawthrop, Tom. 2004. "Cuba Sells Its Medical Expertise." *BBC News.* http://gndp.cigb.edu.cu/News%20BBC%20NEWS%20&%20Cuban%20Biotechnology.htm (accessed 25 April 2004).

Finlayson, Belinda, Jennifer Dixon, Sandra Meadows, and George Blair. 2002a. "Mind the Gap: The Extent of the NHS Nursing Shortage." *British Medical Journal* 325:538–41.

——. 2002b. "Mind the Gap: The Policy Response to the NHS Nursing Shortage." *British Medical Journal* 325:541–44.

Fischman, Josh. 2002. "Nursing Wounds." *U.S. News & World Report,* June 17, 54–55.

Fletcher, Marla. 2002. "Nursing by the Numbers." *Canadian Nurse* 98 (8): 14–16.

Gage, Heather M., Rosemary Pope, and Fiona Lake. 2002. "Nurses' Loyalty May Be Underestimated." *British Medical Journal* 325:1362.

Gaither, Chris. 2000. "South Africa's Latest Cuban Import: Doctors." *South Africa 2000.* http://journalism.berkeley.edu/projects/safrica/adapting/cuban.html (accessed 7 May 2005).

Galvez Tan, Jaime Z. 2003. "Realities and Challenges for the Global Nursing Community." *Philippine Journal of Nursing* 73 (1–2): 8–10.

Gamble, Debi A. 2002. "Filipino Nurse Recruitment as a Staffing Strategy." *Journal of Nursing Administration* 32 (4): 175–77.

GATSwatch. 2004. "What Is GATS?" http://www.gatswatch.org.

Ghose, Ajit K. 2003. *Jobs and Incomes in a Globalizing World.* Geneva: International Labour Office.

Ghosh, Bimal. 2000. "Return Migration: Reshaping Policy Approaches." In *Return Migration—Journey of Hope or Despair?* edited by Bimal Ghosh. Geneva: International Organization for Migration and United Nations.

Ginsberg, Thomas. 2004. "U.S. to Look into Nurse-Screening Firm." *Philadelphia Inquirer,* January 25.

Gonzales, Angela. 2003. "Hospitals Poised for Growth, but Face Staff Shortages." *Business Journal of Phoenix,* September 2. http://allnurses.com/t43598.html (accessed 7 May 2005).

Gordon, Josh, and David Wroe. 2003. "Plan to Court Overseas Students." *The Age,*

May 12. http://www.theage.com.au/articles/2003/05/11/1052591676224.html (accessed 10 February 2004).

Gordon, Suzanne. 2005. *Nursing against the Odds: How Health Care Cost Cutting, Media Stereotypes, and Medical Hubris Undermine Nurses and Patient Care.* Ithaca, NY: Cornell University Press.

Grzincic, Natasha. 2004. "Modern Heroes, Modern Slaves." *Red Pepper,* April. http://www.redpepper.org.uk/Apr2004/x-Apr2004-Grzincic.html (accessed 7 May 2005).

Hampshire, Mary. 2003. "Home and Away." *Nursing Standard* 17 (20): 18–19.

Hanhel, Robin. 1999. *Panic Rules! Everything You Need to Know about the Global Economy.* Cambridge, MA: South End Press.

HANYS (Healthcare Association of New York State). 2003. *Recruiting Foreign-Educated Nurses and Other Professional Health Care Workers for Work in New York State: Facts and Fallacies.* Rensselaer, New York: HANYS. http://www.hanys.org (accessed 4 January 2004).

Harrison, Sarah, and Christian Duffin. 2003. "Foreign Secretary Urged to Act on Underqualified Staff." *Nursing Standard* 17 (19): 8.

Hawthorne, Lesleyanne. 2001. "The Globalisation of the Nursing Workforce: Barriers Confronting Overseas Qualified Nurses in Australia." *Nursing Inquiry* 8 (4): 213–29.

Hopkins, Mary Elizabeth. 2001. "Critical Condition." *NurseWeek,* March 12. http://www.nurseweek.com/news/features/01–03/shortage.asp (accessed 7 May 2005).

HRW (Human Rights Watch). 2000. "UNFAIR ADVANTAGE—Worker's Freedom of Association in the United States under International Human Rights Standards." *Human Rights Watch,* August. http://www.hrw.org/reports/2000/uslabor/ (accessed 7 May 2005).

Huddart, Jenny, and Oscar F. Picazo. 2003. *The Health Sector Human Resource Crisis in Africa: An Issues Paper.* Washington, DC: United States Agency for International Development.

Hurst, Jeremy, and Luigi Siciliani. 2003. "Tackling Excessive Waiting Times for Elective Surgery: A Comparison of Policies in Twelve OECD Countries." OECD Health Working Paper 6. Paris: Organisation for Economic Co-operation and Development.

ICN (International Council of Nurses). 1996. "Reference Document: Professional and Socio-Economic Welfare Responsibilities Within NNAs." Geneva: ICN.

——. 1999a. "Position Statement: International Trade Agreements." Geneva: ICN.

——. 1999b. "Position Statement: Nurse Retention, Transfer and Migration." Geneva: ICN.

——. 1999c. "Position Statement: Socio-Economic Welfare of Nurses." Geneva: ICN.

——. 2000a. "The ICN Code of Ethics for Nurses." Geneva: ICN. http://www.icn.ch/icncode.pdf (accessed 7 May 2005).

——. 2000b. "Position Statement: Occupational health and safety for nurses." Geneva: ICN. http://www.icn.ch/pshealthsafety00.htm (accessed 7 May 2005).

——. 2001a. "Position Statement: Ethical Nurse Recruitment." Geneva: ICN. http://www.icn.ch/psrecruit01.htm (accessed 7 May 2005).

——. 2001b. "ICN Workforce Forum Overview Paper." Geneva: ICN. http://www.icn.ch/forum2001overview.pdf (accessed 7 May 2005).

——. 2001c. "ICN Constitution." Geneva: ICN. http://www.icn.ch/constitution.htm (accessed 7 May 2005).

——. 2002. "*Career Moves and Migration: Critical Questions.*" Geneva: ICN. http://www.icn.ch/CareerMovesMigangl.pdf (accessed 7 May 2005).

——. 2003a. "Press Release: ICN Offers Guidance on Global Nurse Competencies." February 7. Geneva: ICN. http://www.icn.ch/PR05_03 (accessed 11 March 2004).

——. 2003b. "Forum II Report to CNR: Achieving Alternatives to Nursing Migration." Geneva: ICN. http://www.icn.ch/geneva/CNR_ForumII-Eng.pdf (accessed 7 May 2005).

——. 2003c. "ICN Workforce Forum Data Sheet: Nursing Workforce Profile 2003." Geneva: ICN. http://www.icn.ch/SewDatasheet03.pdf (accessed 7 May 2005).

ILO (International Labour Office). 1992. *Equality of opportunity and treatment between men and women in health and medical services.* Geneva: ILO.

——. 1998. *Terms of employment and working conditions in health sector reforms.* Geneva: ILO.

——. 2005. "ILO/WHO to Develop Joint Guidelines on Health Services and HIV/AIDS." Press release, 19 April. Geneva: ILO.

INO (Irish Nurses Organisation). 2003. "Nursing Shortage has Worsened Resulting in Closure of Beds and Cutbacks in Services." Irish Nurses Organisation press release, December 18. http://www.ino.ie/view_categories.php?doc_id=4008&cat=524 (accessed 11 January 2004).

IOM (International Organization for Migration). 2003a. *World Migration 2003—Managing Migration—Challenges and Responses for People on the Move.* Geneva: IOM.

——. 2003b. *Facts and Figures on International Migration.* Geneva: IOM.

Iredale, Robyn. 2001. "The Migration of Professionals: Theories and Typologies." *International Migration* 39 (5, SI-1): 7–24.

——. 2003. "Accreditation of the Qualifications and Skills of Developing Country Service Providers (Mode 4)." Background paper for Expert Meeting on Market Access Issues in Mode 4. Geneva: United Nations Conference on Trade and Development.

IRIN (Integrated Regional Information Network). 2004. "South Africa: Impact of HIV/AIDS on health sector is severe, says study." *U.N. Integrated Regional Information Network,* March 26. http://www.irinnews.org/report.asp?ReportID=40270&SelectRegion= Southern_Afri (accessed 7 May 2005).

Islam, Tabibul. 2002. "Bangladesh Considers Exporting Women, for Foreign Exchange." *South Asia Tribune,* no 11 (September 30–October 6). http://www.satribune.com/archives/sep30_oct06_02/opinion_bangladeshwomen.htm (accessed 7 May 2005).

——. 2003. "Ban or No Ban, Women Workers Leave Home." IPS-Inter Press Service. http://www.ipsnews.net/migration/stories/ban2.html (accessed 7 May 2005).

Janofsky, Michael. 2002. "Shortage of Nurses Spurs Bidding War in Hospital Industry." *New York Times,* May 28. http://www.pef.org/nurses/shortage_of_nurses_spurs_bidding_war.htm (accessed 5 February 2004).

JCAHO (Joint Commission on Accreditation of Healthcare Organizations). 2002. *Health Care at the Crossroads: Strategies for Addressing the Evolving Nursing Crisis.* Washington, DC: JCAHO.

Jordan, Kate. 2000. "Overseas Students in Australia." Background briefing, Radio National, Australia. http://www.abc.net.au/rn/talks/bbing/stories/s108907.htm (accessed 7 May 2005).

Jourdan, Alain. 2003. "La Haute-Savoie met ses infirmières sous perfusion." *Tribune de*

Genève, October 23. http://www.swissdox.ch/index.fr.html (accessed 23 October 2003).

Kai Tiaki Nursing. 2002. "How to Keep Nurses in Nursing." *Kai Tiaki Nursing New Zealand,* July, 8.

Kenny, Craig. 2002. "Call for New Rules on Hiring from Abroad." *Nursing Times* 98 (50): 3.

King, Russell. 2000. "Generalizations from the History of Return Migration." In *Return Migration—Journey of Hope or Despair?* edited by Bimal Ghosh, 7–55. Geneva: International Organization for Migration and United Nations.

Kingma, Mireille. 1999. "Discrimination in Nursing." *International Nursing Review* 46 (3): 87–90.

——. 2001a. "Nursing Migration: Global Treasure Hunt Or Disaster in the Making?" *Nursing Inquiry* 8 (4): 205–12.

——. 2001b. "The Emerging Global Nursing Shortage." Fact sheet. Geneva: International Council of Nurses.

——. 2003. "Economic Incentive in Community Nursing: Attraction, Rejection Or Indifference?" *Human Resources for Health* 1(2): 1–21. http://www.human-resources -health.com/content/1/1/2 (accessed 7 May 2005).

Kisken, Tom. 2004. "Nurses in High Demand: Bonuses, Perks Are Not Enough to Meet Need for New Nurses." *Ventura County Star,* January 4. http://www.msnbc .msn.com/id/3870095 (accessed 11 January 2004).

Kochubka, Gary, Juan J. Flores, Ingrid Amezquita, Cesar Fernandez, and Maria Tapia. 2002. "Mexican Financial Future Flows Weathering Difficult Economic Times." In *Structured Finance.* New York: Standard & Poor's.

Kosel, Keith, and Tom Olivio. 2002. "The Business Case for Work Force Stability." 2002 VHA Research Series 7. https://www.vha.com/research/public/stability.pdf (accessed 7 May 2005).

La Trobe University Faculty of Health Sciences. 2004. "School of Nursing and Midwifery International Programs." http://www.latrobe.edu.au/nursing/ bundoora/son/internat.html (accessed 5 January 2004).

Larson, Jennifer. 2004. "INS Provides Guidance on Foreign Nurse Visas." *NurseZone,* January 5. http://www.nursezone.com/International/NursingInUS.asp ?articleID=9870 (accessed 5 January 2004).

Lewis, Edith P. 2002. "The Rights of Muslims." *American Journal of Nursing* 102 (3): 13.

Lewis, Steven J. 2002. "Retaining Nurses in the NHS: Extent of Shortage Will Be Known Only When Nurses Spend All Their Time Nursing." *British Medical Journal* 325:1362.

Liese, Bernhard, Nathan Blanchet, and Gilles Dussault. 2003. "Background Paper: The Human Resource Crisis in Health Services in Sub-Saharan Africa." Washington, DC: World Bank.

Lindsay, David. 2003/4. "Fijian RNs in Townsville." *Australian Nursing Journal* 11 (6): 45.

Lovell, Jeremy. 2004. "WTO Official Sees No Chance to End Doha This Year." Reuters, February 23.

Lowell, B. Lindsay, and Allan Findlay. 2002. "Migration of Highly Skilled Persons from Developing Countries: Impact and Policy Responses—Synthesis Report." *International Migration Papers,* no. 44. Geneva: International Labour Office.

Macan-Markar, Marwaan. 2003. "Migrant Workers' Convention Not a Magic

Solution." IPS-Inter Press Service. http://www.ipsnews.net/migration/stories/convention.html (accessed 7 May 2005).

Maiden, Samantha. 2003. "Foreign Students Worth $5.2bn a Year." *Australian*, 23 December. http://www.theaustralian.news.com.au/printpage/0,5942,8241486,00.html (accessed 10 February 2004).

Mann, Judy. 1987. "Curing the Nursing Shortage." *Washington Post*, April 3, C3.

Martin, Philip L. 2003a. *Highly Skilled Labor Migration: Sharing the Benefits*. Geneva: International Institute for Labour Studies.

——. 2003b. *Sustainable Migration Policies in a Globalizing World*. Geneva: International Institute for Labour Studies.

——. 2003c. "GATS and Migration." Background Paper for Expert Meeting on Market Access Issues in Mode 4. Geneva: United Nations Conference on Trade and Development.

Martineau, Tim, Karola Decker, and Peter Bundred. 2002. *Briefing Note on International Migration of Health Professionals: Levelling the Playing Field for Developing Country Health Systems*. Liverpool: Liverpool School of Tropical Medicine.

Mason, Diana J. 2002a. "Do Nurses Really Tolerate Diversity?" *American Journal of Nursing* 102 (3): 7.

——. 2002b. "MD-RN: A Tired Old Dance." *American Journal of Nursing* 102 (6): 7.

Mattoo, Aaditya. 2003. "Introduction and Overview." In *Moving People to Services*, edited by Aaditya Mattoo and Antonia Carzaniga, 1–19. Washington, DC: World Bank.

Mcgarvie, Lindsay. 2004. "The NHS Slaves." http://www.sundaymail.co.uk/news/content_objectid=13975586_method=full_sitei(accessed 7 May 2005).

Mejia, Alfonso. 2004. "Migration of Physicians and Nurses: A World Wide Picture." *Bulletin of the World Health Organization* 82 (8): 626–30.

Merckling, Nicolas. 2003a. "Il est inacceptable que Genève ne forme pas le nombre d'infirmières dont elle a besoin." *Le Temps* (Geneva), August 9. http://www.letemps.ch/ (accessed 7 May 2005).

——. 2003b. "La France désarmée face à l'exode de ses infirmières." *Le Temps* (Geneva), October 7, 11.

Mfula, Chris. 2003. "Nurses Brain Drain Shocker!" *Times of Zambia*, December 22. http://allafrica.com/stories/printable/200312220621.html (accessed 3 January 2004).

Milholland, D. Kathy. 2000. *Telenursing, Telehealth: Nursing and Technology Advance Together*. Geneva: International Council of Nurses.

Minton, Anna. 1998. "Nurses Are on Similar Pay to Toilet Cleaners." *Nursing Standard* 12 (39): 9.

Moore, Jean, Sandra McGinnis, Robert Martiniano, and Tracey Contenelli. 2005. "Foreign-Trained Registered Nurses in the United States." Forthcoming.

Mulholland, Helene. 2002a. "Fair Play for Foreign Nurses." *Nursing Times* 98 (36): 8–9.

——. 2002b. "Agencies Failing to Recruit Ethically despite Government Guidelines." *Nursing Times* 98 (46): 3.

——. 2003. "Plan to Train Indian Nurses as RMNs Then Bring Them to UK." *Nursing Times* 99 (25): 4.

——. 2004. "Reid Reneges on Overseas Staff Pledge." *Guardian*, July 26. http://society.guardian.co.uk/NHSstaff/story/0,,1269447,00.html (accessed 7 May 2005).

NCSBN (National Council of State Boards of Nursing). 2003. "Frequently Asked Questions about International NCLEX[(R)] Administration." Chicago: NCSBN.

——. 2004. "About NCSBN." http://www.ncsbn.org/about/index.asp (accessed 7 May 2005).

Nelson, Sioban. 2001. *Say Little Do Much—Nursing, Nuns, and Hospitals in the Nineteenth Century.* Philadelphia: University of Pennsylvania Press.

Nielson, Julia. 2003a. "Labor Mobility in Regional Trade Agreements." In *Moving People to Services,* edited by Aaditya Mattoo and Antonia Carzaniga, 93–112. Washington, DC: World Bank.

——. 2003b. "Service Providers on the Move: Mutual Recognition Agreements." Working Paper for OECD Trade Committee. Paris: Organisation for Economic Co-operation and Development.

Nielson, Julia, and Daria Taglioni. 2003. "A Quick Guide to the GATS and Mode 4." Background paper for the OECD-World Bank-IOM Seminar on Trade and Migration. Paris: OECD Trade Directorate.

Nolen, Stephanie. 2004. "Swaziland's AIDS Rate Leads World" *Globe and Mail* (Toronto), March 24.

NS (Nursing Standard). 2003. "NSH to Investigate Impact of International Recruitment." *Nursing Standard* 18 (12): 9.

NT (Nursing Times). 2001. "Poor Management Is Major Reason for Quitting." *Nursing Times* 97 (35): 4.

——. 2002. "NMC rejects EU proposals." *Nursing Times* 98(30): 5.

——. 2003a. "NI Nurses Fear That Foreign Staff May Be First in Queue for Jobs." *Nursing Times* 99 (4): 5.

——. 2003b. "Legal Doubt Cast on Overseas Screening." *Nursing Times* 99 (10): 4.

——. 2003c. "Skilled Overseas Nurse Used As Cleaner." *Nursing Times* 99 (15): 5.

——. 2003d. "DoH Must Play by Its Own Rules on Overseas Recruitment." *Nursing Times* 99 (28): 13.

O'Dowd, Adrian. 2002. "Surveys Reveal That Younger Nurses Want to Leave the NHS." *Nursing Times* 98 (45): 2.

OECD (Organisation for Economic Co-operation and Development). 2002a. "OECD Publishes for the First Time Statistics on the Direction of Trade in Services." August 18. From Services Industries Trends website. http://www.sitrends.org/facts/figure.asp?FIGURE_ID=82 (accessed 7 May 2005).

——. 2002b. *International Migration of Physicians and Nurses: Causes, Consequences and Health Policy Implications.* Paris: OECD.

——. 2003. *La mobilité internationale des professionelles de la santé: Evaluation et enjeux à partir du cas Sud-africain.* Paris: OECD.

——. 2004a. *The International Mobility of Health Professionals: An Evaluation and Analysis Based on the Case of South Africa.* Paris: OECD.

——. 2004b. "About Services Sector." http://www.oecd.org/about/0,2337,en_2649_34239_1_1_1_1_1,00.html (accessed 7 May 2005).

Omeri, Akram, and Kerry Atkins. 2002. "Lived Experiences of Immigrant Nurses in New South Wales, Australia: Searching for Meaning." *International Journal of Nursing Studies* 39:495–505.

Opiniano, Jeremaiah M. 2002a. "Five OFWs Rescued from UK Private Nursing Home." http://cyberdyaryo.com/features/f2002_0325_04a.htm (accessed 7 May 2005).

——. 2002b. "Over 100 Pinoy Nurses Exploited in UK Private Nursing Homes." http://cyberdyaryo.com/features/f2002_0325_04.htm (accessed 5 January 2004).

———. 2003. "Migration Part of Being a Nurse—Study." http://www.cyberdyaryo
.com/features/f2003_0402_04.htm (accessed 7 May 2005).

O'Sullivan, Anne. 2001. "Statement for the Governmental Affairs Subcommittee on
Oversight of Government Management, Restructuring, and the District of
Columbia on Addressing Direct Care Staffing Shortages." http://nursingworld
.org/gova/federal/legis/testimon/2001/govaref.htm.

Overland, Martha Ann. 2005. "A Nursing Crisis in the Philippines." *Chronicle*
(Manila), January 7. http://chrdonicle.com/weekly/v51/i18/18a04601.htm
(accessed 7 January 2005).

Padarath, Ashnie, Charlotte Chamberlain, David McCoy, Antoinette Ntuli, Mike
Rowson, and Rene Loewenson. 2003. "Health Personnel in Southern Africa:
Confronting Maldistribution and Brain Drain." Equinet Discussion Paper, no. 4.
Harare: Equinet.

Parish, Colin. 2003. "Employ More Nurses and Stop Thousands of Deaths." *Nursing
Standard* 17 (42): 5.

Parris, Janey. 2001. "Keynote Address to Technical Meeting on 'Managed Migration of
Skilled Nursing Personnel.'" *Jamaican Nurse* 39 (1&2): 4–7.

Payne, Linda. 2003. "Differing Viewpoints on the Issue of Overseas Nurses." *Nursing
Times* 99 (13): 15.

Pearce, Lynne. 2003. "A Question of Respect." *Nursing Standard* 17 (45): 14–16.

Penn Nursing. 2004. "Study Abroad." University of Pennsylvania. http://www
.nursing.upenn.edu/admissions/undergrad/options/study_abroad.asp (accessed
7 May 2005).

Petros, Nontyatyambo. 2003. "State, Unions Dispute Holds Up Health Fund."
December 10. http://allafrica.com/stories/200312100169.html (accessed 15
December 2003).

Pinder, Janet M. 2002. "People Starting Nurse Training Should Think Again." *British
Medical Journal* 325:1362.

PNB Trust Banking Group. 2004. "Trust Services." Philippine National Bank.
http://www.pnb.com.ph/trustservicescontent.asp (accessed 7 May 2005).

Power, Jonathan. 2004. "Rethinking the Work Force: Europe Can No Longer Rely on
Immigrant Workers." *International Herald Tribune*, February 19, 6.

PSI (Public Services International). 1997. *International Trade Agreements and Trade
Unions.* Ferney-Voltaire, France: PSI.

Ratha, Dilip. 2003. "Workers' Remittances: An Important and Stable Source of
External Development Finance." In *Global Development Finance 2003—Striving for
Stability in Development Finance,* 157–75. Washington, DC: World Bank.

RCN (Royal College of Nursing). 2002. "Internationally Recruited Nurses Pay Up to
£2,000 to Care for Patients." London: Royal College of Nursing. April 22
http://www.rcn.org.uk/news/display.php?ID=46&area=Press (accessed 7 May
2005).

———. 2003. "Nursing Shortages." Fact sheet. London: Royal College of Nursing.

Ryan, Caroline. 2003. "NHS Is 'Chronically Racist.'" BBC News, April 29. http://
newsvote.bbc.co.uk/mpapps/pagetools/print/news.bbc.co.uk/1/hi/health/2986
(accessed 7 May 2005).

SADC (Southern African Development Community). 2001. "Statement by SADC
Health Ministers on Recruitment of Health Personnel by Developed Countries."
SADC http://www.doh.gov.za/department/sadc/docs/pr/pr0609–01.html
(accessed 7 May 2005).

Salt, John. 2001. "The Business of International Migration." In *International Migration into the 21st Century*, edited by M. A. B. Siddique, 86–108. Cheltenham, UK: Edward Elgar.

Santiago, Maita. 2003. "Overseas Filipinos Targets of SARS-Related Discrimination." *Women's Health News and Issues*, May 3. http://www.cwhn.ca/hot/news/sars -target.html (accessed 26 February 2004).

Sarpong, Sam. 2002. "African Nurses Face Discrimination." *NEWS from AFRICA*, December. http://italy.peacelink.org/newsfromafrica/articles/art_798.html (accessed 7 May 2005).

Scottish Executive. 2004. "AIDS/HIV Infected Health Care Workers: Guidance on the Management of Infected Health Care Workers and Patient Notification." Health and Community Care, Scottish Executive Publications. March 28. http://www.scotland .gov.uk/library5/health/ahhc-04.asp (accessed 7 May 2005).

Shevel, Adele. 2003. "Hospitals Offer Incentives in a Bid to Keep Their Staff." http:// new.hst.org.za/news/index.php/20030207 (accessed 7 May 2005).

Sison, Marites. 2002. "Exodus of Nurses Grows, Health System Feels Effect." Inter Press Service. May 8. http://cyberdyaryo.com/features/f2002_0508_04.htm (accessed 5 January 2004).

Slavery [pseud.]. 2003. "A Nurse's Experience." *Nursing Update*, October, 4–5.

Sochalski, Julie. 2002. "The Changing Picture of Hospital Nurses." *American Journal of Nursing* 102 (5): 93–94.

Sochalski, Julie, Sara Ross, and Daniel Polsky. 2003. "Model of the International Migration of Nurses—A Report for the World Health Organization and the International Council of Nurses." Unpublished.

SouthAfrica.info. 2004. "Transforming the Health Sector." http://www.southafrica .info/ (accessed 7 May 2005).

Spencer, Chris. 2003/4. "Nursing Abroad Broadens Horizons." *Kai Tiaki Nursing New Zealand*, December/January, 14–15.

Stalker, P. 2000. *Workers without Frontiers: The Impact of Globalization on International Migration*. Geneva: International Labour Office.

Stephens, Florence. 2003. "London's Nursing Staff Shortages Are No Surprise." *Nursing Times* 99 (24): 14.

Stewart, Michael. 1998. "Texas Nurse a Leader in Uncovering Visa Scam." American Nurses Association SNA Spotlight. http://nursingworld.org/tan/98marapr/ spotligh.htm (accessed 7 May 2005).

Stiglitz, Joseph E. 2002. *Globalization and Its Discontents*. New York: W. W. Norton. http://www.wwnorton.com/catalog/spring/03/032439excerpt.htm (accessed 12 August 2004).

Stilwell, Barbara, Khassoum Diallo, Pascal Zurn, Mario R. Dal Poz, Orvill Adams, and James Buchan. 2003. "Developing Evidence-Based Ethical Policies on the Migration of Health Workers: Conceptual and Practical Challenges." *Human Resources for Health* 1 (8): 1–19. http://www.human-resources-health.com/content/1/1/8 (accessed 7 May 2005).

Stone, Lauren, and Jennifer Hill. 2003. "Blu-Chip Global Job Connection, Inc Responds to Severe Nurse Shortage in US." http://bluchip.com/press.htm.

Taylor, Sofi. 2003. "UNISON to the Rescue!" *Networking Works, Newsletter of the UNISON Scotland Overseas Nurses Network* 1:3.

Times of India. 2000. "About Remit2India.com." http://www.timesofmoney.com/ remittance/jsp/aboutRemit.jsp (accessed 7 May 2005).

Trossman, Susan. 2002. "The Global Reach of the Nursing Shortage." *American Journal of Nursing* 102 (3). http://www.nursingworld.org/AJN/2002/mar/Issues.htm (accessed 11 January 2004).

UN ECLAC (United Nations Economic Commission for Latin America and the Caribbean). 2003. *Emigration of Nurses from the Caribbean: Causes and Consequences for the Socio-Economic Welfare of the Country: Trinidad and Tobago—A Case Study.* Port-of-Spain, Trinidad and Tobago: UN ECLAC.

UNAIDS/WHO. 2004. "AIDS Epidemic Update." Geneva: United Nations Joint Programme on HIV/AIDS. December.

UNCTAD (United Nations Conference on Trade and Development). 1997a. *International Trade in Health Services: Difficulties and Opportunities for Developing Countries.* Background Note for Trade and Development Board, June 1997. Geneva: UNCTAD.

——. 1997b. *Report of the Expert Meeting on Strengthening the Capacity and Expanding Exports of Developing Countries in the Services Sector: Health Services.* Report for Trade and Development Board, November 1997. Geneva: UNCTAD.

UNHCHR (United Nations High Commission on Human Rights). 2003. "Convention on Protection of Rights of Migrant Workers to Enter into Force Next July." Press Release. March 19. http://www.unhchr.ch/huricane/huricane.nsf/view01/B87E9E85C7147498C1256CEF00385E(accessed 7 May 2005).

University Public Relations. 2001. "Professor 'Nurses' New Team in China." *Currents* 29 (14). University of Rochester. http://www.rochester.edu/pr/Currents/V29/V29N14/story08.html (accessed 7 May 2005).

US Census Bureau. 2000. "U.S. Population: The Basics." *Census 2000.* Washington, DC: U.S. Census Bureau.

US HHS/HRSA/BHPR. 2002. "U.S. Population: The Basics." *Census 2000.* Washington, DC: U.S. Census Bureau.

Volqvartz, Josefine. 2005. "The Brain Drain." *The Guardian,* March 11.

Vujicic, Marko, Pascal Zurn, Khassoum Diallo, Orvill Adams, and Mario R. Dal Poz. 2004. "The Role of Wages in the Migration of Health Care Professionals from Developing Countries." *Human Resources for Health* 2 (3): 1–14.

Wayne, Anne. 2004. "Welcome to Zimbabwe's NHS: Where the Hospital Curtains Are Used for Bandages and Anadin Is Often the Only Drug Left." *Sunday Telegraph* (London), January 25:30.

Webber, Nancy. 2000. "Spread the Word: Safe RN Staffing Saves Lives." *Report—The Official Newsletter of the New York State Nurses Association* October. http://allnurses.comt48301-html (accessed 3 January 2004).

WHO (World Health Organization). 2003. *The World Health Report 2003.* Geneva: WHO.

——. 2004a. "Recruitment of Health Workers from the Developing World." Report to the executive board. Geneva: WHO.

——. 2004b. "International Migration of Health Personnel: A Challenge for Health Systems in Developing Countries." Draft resolution, World Health Assembly. Geneva: WHO.

Wickramasekara, Piyasiri. 2003. "Policy Responses to Skilled Migration: Retention, Return and Circulation." In *Perspectives on Labour Migration* 5E. Geneva: International Labour Office.

Willetts, Annie, and Tim Martineau. 2004. *Ethical International Recruitment of Health Professionals: Will Codes of Practice Protect Developing Country Health Systems?* Liverpool: Liverpool School of Tropical Medicine. http://www.liv.ac.uk/lstm/research/documents/codesofpracticereport.pdf (accessed 7 May 2005).

Winters, A. L., T. L. Walmsley, Z. K. Wang, and R. Grynberg. 2002. *Negotiating the Liberalisation of the Temporary Movement of Natural Persons.* London: Centre for Economic Policy Research.

WMA (World Medical Association). 2003. "The World Medical Association Statement on Ethical Guidelines for International Recruitment of Physicians." May. http://www.wma.net/e/policy/e14.htm (accessed 7 May 2005).

Woodward, David, Nick Drager, Robert Beaglehole, and Debra Lipson. 2002. "Globalization, Global Public Goods, and Health." In *Trade in Health Services: Global, Regional, and Country Perspectives,* edited by Nick Drager and Cesar Vieira, 3–11. Washington, DC: Pan American Health Organization.

World Bank. 2003. "Foreign Investment, Remittances Outpace Debt as Sources of Finance for Developing Countries: World Bank." News release, April 2. http://web.worldbank.org/WBSITE/EXTERNAL/NEWS/0,,contentMDK:20102119~menuPK:3446(accessed 7 May 2005).

WTO (World Trade Organization). 1995. *General Agreement on Trade in Services.* Annex 1B of the Uruguay Round Agreements, Final Act. Geneva: WTO.

——. 1998a. "WTO Adopts Disciplines on Domestic Regulation for the Accountancy Sector." WTO press release, December 14. http://www.wto.org/english/news_e/pres98_e/pr118_e.htm (accessed 7 May 2005).

——. 1998b. "Disciplines on Domestic Regulation in the Accountancy Sector." Adopted by the Council for Trade in Services on December 14. http://docsonline.wto.org/gen_search.asp (accessed 7 May 2005).

——. 2004a. "GATS: Fact and Fiction—Misunderstandings and Scare Stories." http://www.wto.org/english/tratop_e/serv_e/gats_factfictionfalse_e.htm (accessed 7 May 2005).

——. 2004b. "The General Agreement on Trade in Services (GATS): Objectives, Coverage and Disciplines." http://www.wto.org/english/tratop_e/serv_e/gatsqa_e.htm (accessed 7 May 2005).

Xu, Yu. 2003. "Are Chinese Nurses a Viable Source to Relieve the US Nursing Shortage?" *Nursing Economics* 21 (6): 269–74, 279. http://www.medscape.com/viewarticle/465919 (accessed 7 May 2005).

Zachary, Gary. 2001. "Call Them the Ghost Wards." *Wall Street Journal,* January 24.

Index

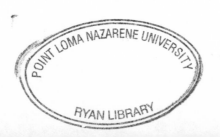